The Psychological After-Effects of Covid

This comprehensive resource provides a one-stop information repository, exploring all psychological aspects of COVID-19. It documents the after-effects of the Covid pandemic, and how it transformed India as a society and its citizens as individuals. The book covers the psycho-social impact on society and individuals and our collective behaviour, as well as coping strategies and interventions and how lessons learned will help in preparedness for the future.

Including case studies and the latest research, this book examines how psycho-social paradigms changed as a result of the pandemic, and left their watermark on the human psyche. It also explores the coping strategies adopted to deal with this common aggressor and how the techniques varied in accordance with social, cultural, and geographical factors. The final chapters offer new insights for the future, highlighting the psychological infrastructure required, the type of preparedness and handling strategies necessary to mitigate the impact of any future biogenic pandemics.

Combining theory and practical application, it will be valuable reading for academics and researchers as well as practising psychologists, clinical psychologists, and law-makers who are concerned with mental health.

Dr Uzaina, PhD, CPsychol, is a Practitioner Counselling Psychologist passionate about helping families and neurodiverse children. She holds critical positions as the Research and Psychology Training Lead at Geniuslane in India and the United Kingdom. Additionally, she founded Psyche Vitality and is the co-director of the Association of Child Brain Research and CDC Solutions India. Dr Uzaina's expertise lies in conducting autism diagnostic assessments and providing essential counselling and support to families. With nearly a decade of experience, she has dedicated herself to offering short-term and long-term counselling and psychotherapy services to adolescents, women, and families. She remains actively engaged in continuous research audits, furthering her commitment to advancing the field of psychology. She also takes great pride in delivering comprehensive training programs to psychology trainees, sharing her knowledge and expertise with the next generation of professionals.

Dr Rajesh Verma is an Assistant Professor and student of Psychology at Feroz Gandhi Memorial Government College Adampur, Haryana. He is an air veteran, academic gold medalist and completed his doctorate from MD University Rohtak. As a report writer, he worked on a DST-funded project on cognitive preparedness. His area of interest lies in indigenous psychology, cognitive psychology, social psychology, psychometrics, organising academic events, and content writing. Recently he organised the ICSSR-sponsored National Conference on "Bhagavad Gita: An Eternal Repository of Multi-disciplinary Lessons for Mankind". He is currently involved in editing a book entitled, "Exploring the Psycho-Social Impact of Covid-19 Global Perspectives on Behaviour, Interventions and Future Directions (Responses)", slated to be published by Routledge. He is tech-savvy, uploads psychology curriculum content-specific videos, and writes blogs regularly. He loves to interact with students.

Dr Ruchi Pandey, PhD, MACP, serves as an Assistant Lecturer at Government Degree College, where she is passionately dedicated to transforming the educational landscape for young women in semi-rural areas and colleges. Her academic journey reflects a remarkable trajectory of achievement, marked by excellence and leadership. As a standout student, Dr Pandey earned the distinction of being the Best Outgoing Student and Topper of her cohort during her undergraduate studies at the University of Lucknow's Awadh Girl's Degree College. She continued her academic prowess during her Master's program at Amity University Lucknow, where she similarly excelled. In 2020, Dr Pandey's outstanding abilities were recognised when she was appointed as a Gazetted Officer through the Uttar Pradesh Service Commission. Dr Pandey's expertise lies in the realm of psychology, with a focus on understanding and crafting psychological measures to enhance individual well-being. Her research interests encompass pivotal areas such as self-forgiveness, self-compassion, resilience, positive body image, and self-affirmations. Through her impactful work, she has amassed over 199 citations in her academic career, a testament to the quality and significance of her contributions to the fields of psychology and self-compassion. Driven by a passion for education and a commitment to empowering young women, Dr Ruchi Pandey inspired and made meaningful strides in her efforts to create positive change in society.

The Psychological After-Effects of Covid

Post-Pandemic Complications and Interventions in India

**Edited by
Dr Uzaina and Dr Rajesh Verma with
Dr Ruchi Pandey**

Routledge
Taylor & Francis Group

LONDON AND NEW YORK

First published 2025
by Routledge
4 Park Square, Milton Park, Abingdon, Oxon OX14 4RN

and by Routledge
605 Third Avenue, New York, NY 10158

Routledge is an imprint of the Taylor & Francis Group, an informa business

British Library Cataloguing-in-Publication Data
A catalogue record for this book is available from the British Library

Library of Congress Cataloging-in-Publication Data
Names: Uzaina, editor. | Verma, Rajesh, editor. | Pandey, Ruchi, editor.
Title: The psychological after-effects of COVID : post-pandemic complications and interventions in India / edited by Dr. Uzaina and Dr. Rajesh Verma with Dr Ruchi Pandey.
Description: Abingdon, Oxon ; New York, NY : Routledge, 2025. | Includes bibliographical references and index.
Identifiers: LCCN 2024010492 (print) | LCCN 2024010493 (ebook) | ISBN 9781032595016 (hardback) | ISBN 9781032595023 (paperback) | ISBN 9781003454984 (ebook)
Subjects: LCSH: Medicine and psychology—India. | COVID-19 Pandemic, 2020—India—Influence. | COVID-19 Pandemic, 2020—India—Psychological aspects.
Classification: LCC R726.5 .P775 2024 (print) | LCC R726.5 (ebook) | DDC 616.001/90954—dc23/eng/20240412
LC record available at https://lccn.loc.gov/2024010492
LC ebook record available at https://lccn.loc.gov/2024010493

ISBN: 9781032595016 (hbk)
ISBN: 9781032595023 (pbk)
ISBN: 9781003454984 (ebk)

DOI: 10.4324/9781003454984

To SARS-CoV-2 who showed a mirror to the humanity and reminded that interfering with nature can lead to existential crisis.

Contents

Figures and tables

Figures

Tables

Contributors

A.V. Abirami is a doctoral research scholar from the Department of English and Cultural Studies. Her research area falls under music and cultural studies. She is a Senior Research Affiliate from the Centre for East Asian Studies, a Former Teaching Assistant and currently serves as a mentor for CAPS at Christ University Bangalore.

Shreyas Babel, a bachelor's student (BS) of Computer Science (University of Michigan, Dearborn, USA) and Data Science and programming (IIT-Madras, India). His main interests are programming, statistics, and data arrangements. He is an efficient programmer. He has a deep interest in Pure Sciences and Mathematics. He has six publications in international journals (SCOPUS & WOS). His interests include listening, learning, and teaching. Quantum computing and AI fascinates him the most and he looks forward to study them in great depth in the near future.

Vineet Gairola is a PhD candidate in Psychology at the Indian Institute of Technology, Hyderabad, where his research focuses on ritual practices and processional worship/journeys of *devī-devtās* (local Hindu deities) in India's Garhwal Himalaya. His research interests focus on cultural psychology, the link between Jung and India, music psychology, psychological perspectives from India, and the correspondence between spirituality, psychopathology, and analytical psychology. He is the winner of the Emerging Psychologists' Programme of the International Congress of Psychology (ICP, Prague); Emerging Scholar Award 2024 from the Religion in Society Research Network, USA; Student Diversity Award 2023 from APA (Division 29); APS Student Grant 2023 from the Association for Psychological Science (APS), USA; the Emerging Scholar Award 2023 from the Religion in Society Research Network, USA; the Excellence in Research Award 2022 by IIT Hyderabad; the Stephen Mitchell Award given by APA (Division 39); the Psychoanalytic Research Exceptional Contribution Award by the International Psychoanalytic Association (IPA); the Student Research Award from APA (Division 36); and the Asian Student Membership Scholarship from the Association for Nepal and Himalayan Studies (ANHS), USA.

Catherine Gomes holds a postgraduate degree in Neuropsychology. Her research spans across cognitive, neuropsychological, developmental, and social psychology. Using eye tracking, she has previously explored the interplay between digital environments and cognitive processes like decision-making. Proficient in conducting neuropsychological assessments, she also delves into studying neurodevelopmental disorders. Catherine's work unravels the complexities of the human mind amid contemporary societal influences.

Mehar Gupta is currently working as a Teaching Assistant in the field of Psychology and has pursued her post-graduation in Psychosocial and Clinical Studies from Ambedkar University, Delhi. With a strong foundation in psychological theories and research methods, she is committed to providing guidance and assistance to students as they navigate through their coursework. She is passionate about fostering a stimulating learning environment and helping students develop critical thinking skills. As a researcher, she has worked in the field of exploring the phenomenology and the complexities involved with individuals diagnosed with mental health disorders.

Nudrat Jahan is working as an Associate Professor in the Department of Psychology, School of Humanities, K. R. Mangalam University, and Gurugram. She has completed her PhD degree in Psychology from Aligarh Muslim University on effectiveness of SSRI, CBT and counselling in treatment of OCD. Her major area of interest is community mental health. She is also associated as a social scientist with Ethical Committees and Institutional Review Board of various Government and private medical colleges. As an active researcher she had worked on national and internal projects and published various papers in reputed national and international journals.

Harshita Jha is currently working as an Assistant Professor, Psychology at The NorthCap University, Gurugram, Haryana. She completed her Masters in Psychology from Indraprastha College for Women (Delhi University) in 2016. She holds a bachelor's degree in Psychology from Lady Shri Ram College for Women (Delhi University). Additionally, she holds a postgraduate diploma in guidance and counselling from Jamia Millia and Islamia. Harshita has previously worked as a research fellow in the field of Military Psychology, at the Defence Institute of Psychological Research (DRDO, New Delhi). In addition, she was engaged with the All India Institute of Medical Sciences (New Delhi) in the capacity of Field Investigator for the project Longitudinal Aging Study of India (Harmonized Diagnostic Assessment Tool for Dementia). Her primary interest areas include Social Psychology, Environmental Psychology, and Indian Psychology. She is especially interested in applying psychological theories and concepts to public policy.

Navkiran Kalsi is currently working as an Assistant Professor, Department of Clinical Psychology, Faculty of Behavioural & Social Sciences, Shree Guru Gobind Singh Tricentenary University, Gurugram, Haryana. She has worked at the National Institute of Mental Health and Neurosciences (NIMHANS,

Bangalore) as a Junior Research Fellow on a project. She, later, received an international scholarship to pursue PhD from La Sapienza- University of Rome (Rome, Italy). Following her PhD. She received a Post-Doctoral Fellowship for her project on Electrophysiological correlates of Problematic Internet Use from the Cognitive Sciences Research Initiative of the Department of Science and Technology of India. She undertook this work at the Brain Mapping Lab of the Department of Psychiatry, AIIMS, New Delhi. Her expertise lies in understanding the role of emotions in cognitive processes in clinical and as well as healthy populations. She has rich experience of working with the Brain Mapping tools like Quantitative EEG, fNIRS, fMRI, and TMS. She is currently establishing a simulation Laboratory in the Department to use Virtual Reality as a tool to understand brain and behaviour and as a tool for psychological interventions.

Anil Kumar is an Assistant Professor (Sociology) and Founder Coordinator, Department of Public Health, Faculty of Humanities and Social Sciences, Shri Ramswaroop Memorial University, Lucknow, India. Dr Kumar has 20 years of teaching and 24 years of research experience. He completed his masters and doctorate from the University of Lucknow, Lucknow, Uttar Pradesh, India. He has published 16 research papers and 4 book chapters. He developed training modules for the health professional working in Uttar Pradesh. He has been a consultant with State Nutrition Mission, Uttar Pradesh. He led the team of the National Family Health Survey-5, for 27 districts of Eastern Uttar Pradesh. Presently he is working on two projects on (a) 'Involvement of NSS Volunteers for Addressing Health Issues with Youth of Degree Colleges' and (b) 'Health Promotion focusing mental Health & Life skills among Youth' funded by the State Innovations in Family Planning Services Project Agency, Lucknow. He is Founder Member Secretary of the Institutional Ethics Committee, SRMU, Lucknow, Assistant Secretary, Ethnographic and Folk Culture Society, Lucknow, and Member, Executive Committee, Baba Ram Karan Das Grameen Vikas Samiti, Gorakhpur.

Jayant Kumar is currently working as Joint Director in the Department of Health and Family Welfare, Govt. of Uttar Pradesh in Devipatan Division of Uttar Pradesh. He has done his bachelor's in Medicine and Surgery (MBBS) in 1989 from Ganesh Shankar Vidyarthi Memorial Medical College (GSVM) Kanpur, Uttar Pradesh. He is having more than 32 years of experience in the field of Public Health and Medicine. Dr Jayant has started his carrier as a Medical Officer in Sultanpur district of Uttar Pradesh. He has worked as a senior medical officer, consultant, senior consultant, additional CMO, CMO, and Joint director in the health department. He had played a key role in monitoring and evaluation of several National Health Programmes in various districts of Uttar Pradesh.

Pradeep Kumar is an Assistant Professor in the Department of Psychology at the Central University of Haryana, India. He has over ten years of teaching experience and has supervised 12 master's dissertations. Currently, he is supervising four PhDs. His areas of expertise include Personality, Psychometrics, and

Mental Abilities. He has published more than 20 research papers in reputed national and international journals.

Sanjay Kumar is presently working with Guru Jambheshwar University of Science & Technology, Hisar and has done his PhD from Central Institute of Psychiatry, Ranchi in 2011. He has authored 2 books, 10 chapters in National and International books, and more than 40 research papers in journals of repute. His thrust areas are Clinical Psychology, Substance Dependence, Psychological Assessment and Psychotherapeutics.

Anita Manglani is currently working as an Assistant Professor, Department of Clinical Psychology, Faculty of Behavioural & Social Sciences, Shree Guru Gobind Singh Tricentenary University, Gurugram, Haryana. She is a strong professional with a Postdoc (ICSSR), PhD (MLSU), NET (UGC), & DCGC (NCERT). She has worked on various projects under RUSA (MHRD), UGC, and Indian Council of Agricultural Research (ICAR). She has various tests and scales, book chapters, research article publications, in different national and international journals. She is awarded with Excellence Award (2019) and Appreciation Award for COVID-19 Service from the District Collector and District Magistrate (2020).

Abhishek Mishra is currently working as a Public Health Specialist, District Surveillance Officer, and District Nodal Officer for Vector Borne Disease in Department of Health and Family Welfare, Govt. of Uttar Pradesh, Ballia District. He has done his bachelor's in Medicine and Surgery (MBBS) in 2011 and later completed postgraduate diploma in maternal and child health, completed two-year Epidemic Intelligence Services training programme from the National Centre for Disease Control, New Delhi. He has done "Masters in Public Health" as well. Dr Mishra has started his carrier as a Junior Resident Doctor in "Guru Gobind Government Hospital Delhi" after working there for a while he has joined "Department of Health and Family Welfare, Govt. of Uttar Pradesh" as a Medical Officer in the year 2012. As a Medical Officer he has worked for monitoring, supervision, and evaluation of various National Health Programmes at district and state levels. He was also part of State Rapid Response Team of Uttar Pradesh (UP) for two years (2017–2018) during this period he investigated, Japanese Encephalitis outbreak in district Bahraich, Dengue outbreak in Lucknow and Varanasi, Malaria outbreak in Bareilly and Badayun. Dr Mishra was one of the early core committee member for "Dastak Abhiyan" conducted by Govt. of Uttar Pradesh for prevention and control of Acute Encephalitis Syndrome and other vector borne disease. Dr Mishra is an empanelled "External Quality Assessor" for public health facilities under National Health System Resource System (NHSRC) a quality division under National Health Mission, Government of India. Dr Mishra has published in peer-reviewed journals and has contributed in making of "Guidance Document on Foodborne Diseases Outbreak Investigation by FSSAI".

Shachi Mishra received her Master of Science in Chemistry from Banasthali University, Banasthali, in 2012 and then PhD from Central Drug Research Institute,

Lucknow in 2019 in Medicinal Chemistry with emphasis on design and synthesis of donor-acceptor based heterocyclic compounds for biological and
diagnostic applications. Dr Mishra joined Post-Graduate Department of Chemistry, Jai Prakash University, Chapra, Bihar in 2018, as Assistant Professor. Her
research interests lie in Medicinal Chemistry, Synthetic Organic Chemistry,
Nanochemistry, design and development of theranostic Fluorescent probes, and
Computational Chemistry. She has published more than ten research papers in
international journals. She has been a Gold medallist in MSc and M.M. Dhar
Memorial distinguished career achievement award, 2019 in Chemical Sciences.

Shalini Mittal earned her PhD in Psychology from Banaras Hindu University,
India. She is currently working as an Assistant Professor at the School of Liberal Arts, Bennett University, India. She is trained in the skill of interviewing
victims of crime and aims to amplify the voices and impact of victims, gender,
and minorities through her research work.

Sneha Mittal is pursuing PhD in Psychology from the Department of Applied
Psychology, Guru Jambheshwar University of Science & Technology, Hisar,
Haryana, India and also currently working as Guest Faculty in the Department
of Psychology, Central University of Haryana, Mahendergarh, Haryana, India.
She has authored 5 book chapters and 12 research papers in journals of repute.

Ms Parul is presently working as an Assistant Professor of Computer Science at
Shaheed Smark Government P.G. College, Faridabad, Haryana. She has more
than ten years of teaching experience. Her research areas are wireless sensors,
database management systems, digital divide, internet of things, artificial intelligence, new media technologies, and women's participation in the technology
area. She has contributed several papers to various journals and presented papers
in national and international conferences. She is a communicator of issues of
ethics and social responsibility among technology users. She has delivered several lectures especially on applications of the internet and artificial intelligence
to students.

Asma Parveen (Chairperson in the Department of Psychology, Aligarh Muslim
University) served in the Psychology department for more than two decades.
She did her postgraduation in both Psychology (with gold medal) and Business
Administration (MBA). Her areas of specialisation are Organisational, Abnormal, and Biopsychology. She has published 32 research papers in journals of
national and international repute, and also wrote 15 chapters in different books.
She has also contributed in the development of study material for PG Diploma
in Guidance and Counseling of Distance and Open Learning program of Jamia
Millia Islamia, New Delhi. She has guided six PhD and two MPhil scholars
successfully. One PDF has also been awarded under her supervision. At present
seven research scholars are pursuing their PhD work under her guidance.

Angela Peter serves as a psychologist at Nirmal Chhaya Complex, a Child Care
Institute operating under the aegis of the Ministry of Women and Child Development. Possessing a master's degree in Lifespan Counselling, Angela specialises

in crisis intervention, particularly Borderline Personality Disorder, ADHD, and Mood Disorders.

Shubham Prasad, an accomplished individual, holds a distinction in his Master's degree in Clinical Psychology from the prestigious SGT University, located in Gurugram, Haryana. Shubham's scholarly pursuits are focused on his deep interest in delving into the intricacies of personality traits, abnormal psychology, and the fascinating psychology that permeates everyday life. He is an Avid Book Reader and Master Visualiser – Imaginator, Amateur Artist and Art Enthusiast and Novitiate in Creative Writing.

Abhay Rabia is a doctoral research scholar in psychology, CHRIST (Deemed to be University). His field of specialisation is in consumer neuroscience. He has had extensive experience in creating research designs and has worked as a teaching assistant, teaching subjects like neuropsychology, cognitive psychology, and so on. He is an assessing editor in the journal of mind and behaviour. He has one scopus-indexed book chapter publication.

Kritika Rastogi currently works as an assistant professor in the Department of Psychology at CHRIST (Deemed to be University) in Delhi, NCR. She has more than seven years of teaching and industry experience. Her areas of interest are positive psychology, counselling psychology, and education psychology. She has extensively worked with school-teachers during her PhD. She has conducted research on topics like mental health, the life satisfaction of teachers, and cooperative learning. She is a certified hypnotherapist.

Shaveta Sachdeva is associated with the School of Management and Liberal Studies, The NorthCap University as an Assistant Professor of Economics. Her areas of expertise include microeconomics, environmental economics, and international economics/business. She has seven years of work experience in academics, research, and administration at institutions of repute. Prior to joining NCU she was associated with the Manav Rachna University as an Assistant Professor. She has also worked with Shree Guru Gobind Singh Tricentenary University and Dayalbagh Educational Institute, Agra. She holds PhD in Economics from Dayalbagh Educational Institute Agra and is NET qualified. She has published research papers/book chapters/articles in various peer-reviewed journals in the area of social sciences and management. She has also presented 20+ research papers at both national and international seminars organised by IIT Roorkee, IIBR Pune, Indus Business Academy Noida and IBS Bangalore, etc. She is also a certified digital teacher by the ICT Academy.

Roma Seraj is working as a guest faculty in the Department of Psychology, Lalit Narayan Mithila University, Bihar, India. She received a doctorate degree from the Psychology Department, Aligarh Muslim University, India. Her research interests lie in clinical and social psychology. She has authored two research papers in a reputed journal from Disabilities and Impairment – an Interdisciplinary Research Journal.

Megha Sharma is a RCI licensed clinical psychologist. She is currently working as Assistant Professor, Department of Clinical Psychology, Faculty of Behavioural & Social Sciences, Shree Guru Gobind Singh Tricentenary University, Gurugram, Haryana. She has worked in AIIMS, Delhi hospital as a clinical psychologist in different departments such as Psychiatry and medicine. She has also served as a faculty in the Department of Clinical Psychology as Assistant Professor at Amity University, Haryana.

Sudha Shashwati is an Assistant Professor in the School of Liberal Studies, UPES, Dehradun. She is also a trainer for mental health capacity building, a comprehensive sexually educator, and a psychotherapist engaged in trans-diagnostic, process-based psychotherapy. Her areas of research interest are gender relations, youth mental health, and cultural studies.

Pavitra Singh is a Research Scholar in the Department of Psychology at the Central University of Haryana, India. Her research interest lies in Indian Psychology and currently she is pursuing PhD on Rajyoga Meditation. She has published four research papers in reputed national and international journals, out of which one is scopus indexed.

Tushar Singh obtained his DPhil in psychology from the University of Allahabad and is currently serving as Assistant Professor at Banaras Hindu University, India. His research focuses on understanding the miseries of and advocation for the rights of gender and social minorities including but not limited to LGBTQ+, abused women, and children. He is also involved in academic administration and is associated with various national and international organisations in various capacities.

Sruthi Suresh is a doctoral research scholar in Psychology at CHRIST (Deemed to be University) examining School Bullying through a socio-ecological framework. In 2018, she completed her Masters in Counseling Psychology and worked as an IB DP Psychology Faculty for the next two years. After joining the PhD program in 2020, she has been an active scholar and engaged with the department as a Research Assistant, Teaching Assistant, Impact Assessment Research Team Lead, and Department Magazine Editor. She writes and presents widely on issues related to child and adolescent mental health, teacher education, and social-emotional learning. She has two Scopus-indexed book chapter publications, and she presently works as a Psychology Educator and TOK Coordinator at the Knowledgeum Academy in Bengaluru.

Ishanpreet Kaur Toor is a PhD scholar in the Department of Psychology at Christ (Deemed to be University). She is pursuing her PhD in behavioural medicine. Her research comprises both Spiritual/Transcendental psychology and health psychology. She has also qualified UGC NET in Psychology. She is also a recipient of a Junior Research Fellowship from the University Grants Commission. She is also trained as a meditation teacher.

Bhawna Tushir is an Assistant Professor of Psychology at Christ University, Delhi-NCR, India with extensive experience in Malviyan and Gandhian Philosophy. She has worked with several universities and organisations as a trainer and consultant. She is committed to providing rigorous and evidence-based research, ensuring that the findings are reliable and contribute to the existing knowledge in the field.

Durgesh Kumar Upadhyay is an Assistant Professor in the Department of Psychology, Mahatma Gandhi Kashi Vidyapith, Varanasi since 2018. Coordinator of one of its first in Uttar Pradesh, Music Therapy Lab/Cell & Research Centre, Dr Upadhyay is also the Visiting Faculty at the Institute for Women Studies, University of Lucknow, Lucknow and Sri Sri University, Odisha. Dr Durgesh has completed his MA in Clinical Psychology from Dev Sanskriti Vishwavidyalaya, Haridwar and DPhil (Psychology) in Music Psychology University of Allahabad, Allahabad. He is a certified Music Therapist and a Vocalist.

Rakesh Verma is presently working as Extension Lecturer at MNS Govt. College Bhiwani, Haryana. He has more than a decade of teaching experience in university and college. He completed his doctorate from Sardar Patel University Anand, Gujrat, India. He is certified and Rehabilitation Council of India registered rehabilitation psychologist. His areas of interest are social psychology, clinical psychology, indigenous psychology, and report writing. He had published research paper in national and international journals and presented papers in conferences. He has one book to his credit. He is an active philanthropist and have expertise in Indian Knowledge Systems.

Sujit Verma is presently working as Postgraduate Teacher of Physical Education in the Department of School Education, Government of Haryana. She obtained her doctorate from Punjabi University, Patiala, Punjab, and masters from the prestigious Lakshmi Bai National Institute of Physical Education (Deemed to be University), Gwalior. She has more than two decades of experience of teaching school, colleges, and university students. She has been a national gold medallist in gymnastics. She has been resource person and delivered invited talks at several institutions. Her interest lies in sports psychology, bio-mechanics, and kinesiology. She is an avid reader and expert in proof reading of manuscripts.

Foreword

COVID-19 has become a household word across the globe, thanks to its audacity in challenging the entirety of humanity. It was no less than the secondary existential crisis that led to overhauling the human approach towards meaningfulness and purpose of life. Its impact forced the world to scramble to contain the spread. The technology that aided the spread came in handy in limiting and finally controlling its unabated psycho-somatic destruction. Humanity was collective in its efforts to grapple with the unprecedented physical health challenges caused by the virus and the intense psychological ones. By virtue of its mode of spread and novelty of structure, it has left an indelible mark on the universal consciousness. As we try to pick up the thread and move through the psychological debris left behind by COVID-19, it is imperative to gather scientific traces to explore and understand the psychological dimension of the COVID-19 era.

With 1.4 billion people and a diverse cultural fabric, India has also not remained untouched by the virus's dirty drive. Though the initial spread was slow and the physical infection rate was low, the psychological infection was as high as in other countries. Even a single addition to the dreaded list of infected and identified people was enough to shiver the psychological spine of the entire India. Against this backdrop, this book, "The Psychological After-Effects of COVID: Post-Pandemic Complications and Interventions in India", serves as a one-stop repository of the handiwork of the virus and human effort to tide over its effects.

The volume has diverse studies that delve deep into the unique experiences of a young nation but old civilisation. The book rightfully starts with an introductory chapter that provides brief and oversight view of the upcoming chapters. It is expected to help in making decision whether to go ahead with the read or not. The chapters align with the book's theme and successfully illustrate how the psychological repercussions transcended multidimensional health challenges. The editors quite intelligently articulated the chapters in a flow, starting the book with a systematic review that included articles that studied the psycho-social consequences of COVID-19 across age groups. The reading flow has been maintained well with the placement of the second chapter, which explores the psycho-social implications of COVID-19 with the application of photovoice techniques. The virus has rendered extensive damage to the psycho-social fabric of society mainly due to the unexpected associated outcomes. The significant psychological impact was a manifestation of anxiety, fear, and depressive symptoms. The fear of the unknown with unknown consequences, and we all were unaware of the possible cure. One of the major gainers during the pandemic was internet. The information seeking is a subset of natural curiosity, which drives humans to discover and invent. A massive demand for the internet to satiate information hunger was witnessed across the sectors. Though the internet has helped in getting things done yet, it has contributed to added anxiety-related symptoms and consequent behaviours. One of the additions was a situation where individuals search the internet for medical conditions. Intentional Internet surfing for self-diagnosis through matching the symptoms is, in trend, intensifying the anxiety manifestation.

To understand the impact and challenges of COVID-19, the third chapter is right fit where data of one of the districts of Uttar Pradesh has been analysed through situational analysis. The figures and facts paints the gory picture of three waves of COVID-19 infection and ensuing causalities. The data shows that the second wave was proved to be more deadly than the first and third wave. It might due to the fact that during the first wave we were extra vigilant and we employed extreme measures while during the third wave the preparedness was adequate and people were immunised, too.

The academic journey through the chapters will shed light on various psychological issues faced by the Indian population, including speculated anticipatory anxiety in social interactions and the development and experience of COVID-19-related anxiety. At the pandemic's peak, the people's trust was at its nadir. Everyone automatically assumed to be the virus carrier. And those who were infected and later recovered were treated as straight out-cast. The mixed feelings added fuel to the experiential anxiety and stigmatisation of the individual. The studies on experiences and impact of COVID-19 on police persons and music professionals were added to understand the reach of the virus. The book weaves personal narratives, scientific research, and coping insights to understand the post-COVID-19 psychological scene in India comprehensively.

Though not demarcated by the editors, the following section deals with coping mechanisms. Individual coping mechanisms play a pivotal role in fostering resilience and recovery. India is the cradle of spirituality and self-exploration. The spirituality that has developed through the thousands of years of experience has permanently seeped into the genetic code of every Indian. The impact of spirituality is visible in the day-to-day behaviour and cultural setting of Indians. The unique behaviour of Indians is that whenever they face any problem, disease, or accident, usually the first reaction is that it must have been the will of God or some supernatural power. The particular and India-specific reaction type can only result from deep spiritual contemplation and total trust dedication. So, it is no surprise to find the last lap of the book with chapters exploring coping strategies modulated with spiritual leanings, such as spiritual disposition, spiritual tourism, and Rajyoga meditation.

As we are at a critical juncture where the natural flow of humanity is gradually getting diverted towards science, we must understand that society is the base of being human. The present state is no less than a crisscross of science, spirituality, and mental health. This book will be expected to be the lighthouse for the travellers in the alleys of policymaking, managing health, developing psychological health infrastructure, curious academicians, researchers, students, and masses. It is the concrete indicator of the psycho-socio resilience of humanity and collective efforts that pop up in the face of existential crisis-like situations. Finally, the last chapter has brilliantly summarised the contents for a quicker glance for the readers.

Humanity is and will have to grapple with uncertainty despite scientific progress. In this context, "The Psychological After-Effects of COVID" stands as an apposite contribution that has attempted to shed light on the dark shadows cast by the COVID-19-led pandemic and light the path with its invaluable inputs. I wish you all the best with your book, and I hope it will help humanity better understand the psychological impact and coping strategies employed by the Indians. I am sure this book will initiate a dialogue to help prepare humankind to deal with pandemic-type adversities and foster universal psychological well-being.

Manas K. Mandal
PhD, FNAPsy
Distinguished Visiting Professor at
Indian Institute of Technology Kharagpur

Preface

My daughter asked me, "Why do we remember bad things?" "Because the memory of bad things is a psychological vaccination that helps in protecting our thought process from contamination and developing abstract resiliency", was my reply. Memories of bad experiences or trauma strengthen our cognition, enhancing cognitive preparedness. My daughter was perplexed by my answer, probably due to technical jargon. Her face seemed to be more confused with minute expressions of artificial surprise. I quickly realised my mistake and explained it to her in simple terms. This event motivated me to collaborate and compile the COVID-19-related memories [bad] in this volume. This book will likely serve the purpose of conveying, connecting, sharing, and contemplating the dreadfulness of SARS-CoV-2.

The unbridled run of coronavirus in the last month of 2019 unfolded a flood of varied challenges for humanity. The virus gained popularity in the name of COVID-19 (Corona Virus Disease 2019), the self-explanatory nomenclature given by WHO. According to WHO, "Viruses are named based on their genetic structure to facilitate the development of diagnostic tests, vaccines and medicines". However, the repercussions of COVID-19 are beyond its usual purpose. COVID-19 is a dread alphanumeric word. Maybe not now, but ask those who lived through the initial phase when nothing was known about the virus except it is the shortest route to death. Maybe not now, but ask those who lived through the initial phase of the COVID-19 tsunami when nothing was known about the virus except it was the shortest and quickest route to death.

"The Psychological After-Effects of COVID: Post-Pandemic Complications and Interventions in India" is a comprehensive exploration of the aftershocks of the pandemic on the mental landscape of India. The book is designed to understand the complexity of often overlooked and underreported outcomes of COVID-19 on the psychological health of the Indian population. The book is destined to shed light on the challenges faced by Indian society on the mental health front. Additionally, it delves deep into the indigenous and standard interventions and coping mechanisms employed by culturally diverse societies based on the solid foundation of values and peace-promoting philosophy. This volume aims to provide a holistic understanding of the psychological aftermath of the pandemic in India.

How a nation with a billion-plus population could brilliantly manage the unprecedented global crisis that unfolded in the biogenic pandemic is a matter of study and emulation. India and the world were unaware of the virus first detected in Wuhan. Along with the physical destruction of lives, the COVID-19-led fear pandemic left an indelible mark on the unsuspecting psyche of human civilisation. The most challenging feature of the COVID-19 virus was its style of "unknown and omnipresent". The joint effort of public and private agencies associated with a resilient society based on pro-social values played a significant buffer in mitigating the impact. Despite unified efforts, the virus was able to infect 45001245 (4.5 crore) Indians, out of which 533293 died (death rate 1.185%) (WHO, 2023). Just as the nukes in Hiroshima and Nagasaki left a trail of longitudinal destruction, COVID-19 ensured the Hiro-Naga nuke saga silently, the psychological after-effects of COVID-19. The impact of COVID-19 was visible in a chain reaction style. Targeting the central gear [human being] of the growth story. In India, the most profound impact of the pandemic was observed on mental health with multifaceted outcomes.

The chapters within this volume cover a wide range of topics, from impact and challenges of COVID-19: A Situational Analysis, speculated anticipatory anxiety of social interactions post-COVID-19, experiences of music professionals during the COVID-19 pandemic, the exploration of psycho-social experiences of college going youth through photovoice, critical analysis of the transactional concept of coping through media during the pandemic, the practice-cum-application of spiritual tourism to tide over the COVID-19 led burnout, *Rajyoga* meditation as an intervention technique for managing negative affect accrued to pandemic, exploration and analysis of spiritual dispositional coping and health hardiness on stress and related illnesses that had developed due to pandemic, the role of psychological capital in dealing with COVID-19 related mental well-being in police personnel and finally a systematic review of 41 articles on psycho-social consequences of COVID-19.

As we are destined to tread the uncertain path ahead, we must acknowledge and address the psychological scars left by COVID-19 and strive with synergy to ensure the comprehensive well-being of humanity. This book is a step towards that goal, and we thank all the contributors who have shared their writings to make this abstract endeavour a tangible reality.

Dr Rajesh Verma

Acknowledgements

At the outset we would like to express our gratitude to all the contributors without which the completion of this research monologue, "The Psychological After-Effects of Covid: Post-Pandemic Complications and Interventions in India" would not have been possible.

We express our deepest thanks to our publisher for believing in the significance of this work and supporting us throughout the publication process. Your guidance and professionalism have been instrumental in shaping this monologue.

We thank Professor Manas K. Mandal, PhD, FNAPsy for forwarding this research monologue.

We thank all the peer reviewers for their insightful feedback and constructive criticism that refined the quality of the contents of this monologue.

We are immensely grateful to our families and friends for their unwavering support, understanding, and encouragement during the countless hours spent researching, writing, and editing this monologue.

We would also like to acknowledge the support of our colleagues, friends, and family members who provided encouragement, understanding, support, and motivation throughout this academic journey. Special thanks to our children for disturbing less during the process.

Thank you, each and every one, for your invaluable contributions and help which has been the driving force behind this endeavour, and we are truly grateful for the opportunity to present this work to the world.

With warm regards,

Editors

Introduction to the Research Monologue

Uzaina, Rajesh Verma, and Ruchi Pandey

World Health Organisation defines coronavirus disease (COVID-19) as an infectious disease caused by the SARS-CoV-2 virus (WHO, 2023). The current statistics about COVID-19 cases in India that have been cured or discharged are 4,44,84,733, and the total number of deaths counts to 5,33,412; total recorded vaccinations are 22,06,782,853 and at present total active cases are 3,368 (MyGov.in., 2024).

Starting with a case study of an 18-year-old boy and his family impacted by the First Wave of COVID-19 in 2020, he was travelling with his friends on his birthday; he was the only son and used to live with his mother and father. Father was diagnosed with liver sclerosis and recently had a liver transplant twice within the previous year. Father suddenly got very sick, and as it was lockdown, no medical doctor agreed to come and see him. Until an ambulance could have been arranged, he took his last breath.

Within the next six months, his mother, who was in her 40s during the third wave of COVID-19, got COVID-19 positive; due to the lack of hospital beds and infrastructure, they stayed at home, thinking they would be able to manage COVID-19 themselves. When the Oxygen Saturation dropped down, the family took her to a private hospital. She was stabilised overnight, then again, her oxygen saturation went down, and the hospital asked them to take her to another hospital. This 18-year-old male from an affluent family reports paying an ambulance driver 50k INR so her mother can be transferred from a private hospital to another government hospital. She was kept there overnight, and in the afternoon, the doctor reported to the boy that she was no more. The boy did the cremation himself, with no family members present, standing at a crossroads in his life where he lost everything to this pandemic. This is just one case out of those 5,33,412 deaths that happened during the COVID-19 pandemic.

In this case study, we have tried to highlight that the pandemic which hit us in late 2019 started a chain of catastrophic psycho-physiological events that have never been seen before or imagined. Not just limited to the physical impact, but it changed the whole canvas of what we used to think normalcy was, leaving its mark on psycho-social, mental health, and financial domains and starting with the

DOI: 10.4324/9781003454984-1

closing of international and domestic travel, with closed domestic borders of the states, causing so much uncertainty and chaos and resulting in so many deaths, losses, indecent of loved ones not being able to say final goodbye to the deceased, and unable to pay their last respect to the death, and not being able to do the last rites. Gradually moving away from the pandemic with the aid of vaccines, awareness, and responsible behaviour across countries, it's still not eradicated.

The pandemic was a challenging phase because of the lockdown breakdown of the healthcare system, but above all this, what kept this country of 1.42 billion people going is a question worth asking (Population of India, n.d). As researchers and psychologists, we needed to document its impact on the masses and the long-term footprints it would leave on the psyche before it was finally eradicated. Through this first series of the research monologue, we, along with the authors, have tried to document the after-effects of the pandemic and how it transformed us as a society and individuals.

The first section starts with a systematic review (SR), reviewing studies on psycho-social consequences. The primary purpose of including SR as the first chapter is to acquaint the reader with the range and size of the impact of COVID-19 on the psychological and social landscape. It primes the reader for further reading and creates an academic curiosity for content types. From the over-and-above analysis of findings in the first chapter, the next chapter provides glimpses of specific cases where the effect of COVID-19 on young students has been explored through the photovoice technique. The scope of the impact of the COVID-19-led pandemic on the general population is possible only when its effect on every strata, specifically the productive population, is studied. The debilitating impact of the highly versatile virus spared none of the population strata. Young students are one of the productive populations studied and included in the second chapter. Though images and pictures have been attracting humanity since the very inception stage and are found to be highly successful in presenting a more convincing paradigm of a situation in the present scroll-and-click age, pictures have become more than relevant. The second chapter rightly captures the present mood of the young population by using the photovoice technique to understand the impact and effect of COVID-19 on their psycho-social profile. The physical treatment and subsequent interventions were discovered with technology, but the significant cause of concern was the development of practical and workable interventions for psychological damage. Significant psychological damage was done through the depressive and anxiety attacks. COVID-19 was so intense in its effect that it was successful in engendering speculated anxiety among the population. People displayed highly speculative and anticipatory anxiety in the sense that they are the next target of COVID-19, where their lungs will be first affected (Wadman et al., 2020), resulting in a drop in oxygen levels. The speculation forced people to purchase electronic gadgets that measure respiratory rate, oxygen saturation level, blood pressure, streaming devices, and pulse meters, among others. Channa et al. (2021) concluded that the demand for wearable devices was risen during the pandemic. However, they are lying unused now but played an essential role in the speculated anxiety during the pandemic.

A critical development during the pandemic was the psychological disturbance parallel to the physical damage done by the virus. Usually, psychological disorders either precede or follow the physical ailment. The COVID-19 case carried the tag of virus-without-known-cure and spread faster than expected through most common means of human interaction. The virus was potent enough to modify the age-old Western greeting style overnight; it was nothing less than watershed modification. The 'fear' [fear of contacting (FoC)] was the fundamental reason for the watershed modification. The FoC led to the development of another psychological issue connected with prejudiced attitudes commonly known as social stigma and public stigma by APA. The severity of COVID-19 led to social stigma, even pushing WHO to issue a page guide for prevention and addressing the social stigma for governments, media, and medical organisations on 24 February 2020. Seyed Alinaghi et al. (2023) reported 22 studies in their SR specifically focused on COVID-19 that led to social stigma. The importance of this social phenomenon was considered covered in the book; hence, it has been addressed in a study in the fifth chapter.

The challenging journey through COVID-19 times infused us with stocktaking of our preparedness for biological disasters that have disastrous psycho-social ramifications in tune with physical issues. One preparatory aspect for dealing with the pandemic is listing, teaching and making the general population aware of coping strategies. The psychological concept of coping is learned and has traces of genetics (non-additive effect of genetics on coping, Dunn & Conley, 2015). The coping strategies tend to vary depending upon several factors such as situation, dispositional traits, problem type, cultural factors, intensity of the problem, and available resources. The book has been based on the Indian population; hence, it is not surprising that most chapters on coping strategies were pinned on the spiritual aspect. India is the world capital of spiritualism and alternative approaches dealing with fundamental questions on the relevance of the existence of human beings. India is dominated by spiritual tourism, where domestic and international tourists visit Indian sites for spiritual tourism.

The seventh chapter investigates how psychological capital influences the mental well-being of police personnel amid the COVID-19 pandemic. It outlines the pandemic's significant impact on global mental and physical health, particularly emphasising the unique challenges faced by law enforcement officers. Psychological capital, encompassing attributes like hope and resilience, emerges as a vital tool for officers to navigate their demanding roles during this crisis. The chapter highlights the positive correlation between psychological capital and mental well-being among police personnel, underscoring specific dimensions like hope as key predictors. It also addresses gender disparities in psychological capital and mental well-being, advocating for targeted support initiatives. Additionally, the chapter suggests practical interventions such as counselling and workload management to promote officers' mental health. It concludes by emphasising the crucial role of psychological capital in enhancing the resilience of police personnel and advocating for further research to inform effective interventions.

The Indian civilisation has developed the most varied and adaptable approaches vis-à-vis human existence. In this context, the book would only be complete if we included the spiritual aspect. Spiritual concepts offer unconditional solace for all situations, even if they offer hope for situations beyond human control. The pandemic engendered excessive stress, which culminated in stress-related issues and unwarranted anxiety. The chapters included in the book address various psychological problems that were handled using spiritual coping mechanisms. One of the unique features of spirituality that makes it successful in addressing multiple psychologically related issues is that it touches almost every aspect of human life and provides sustained cognitive relief. It offers psychological support that makes an individual resilient and mentally efficient enough to handle various crises. Apart from the spirituality-led coping studies, one study on the relaxation technique has been included in the book. The idea behind including this strategy is to familiarise the reader with the effectiveness and procedure of spiritual techniques. Chapter 9 extensively explores the role of Rajyoga meditation in dealing with pandemic-led comprehensive negativism. Rajyoga meditation has been found to have a therapeutic effect on managing psychological disorders; for example, Mehta et al. (2020) found that Rajyoga meditation helped in mitigating the symptoms of OCD. Considering the effectiveness and potency of spiritual mechanisms, including these strategies in the present book was imperative. The last chapter provides an in-depth exploration of how individuals cope with grief and stress amidst the global crisis, focusing on the role of electronic media. It begins by categorising different types of grief and discussing established models of coping, such as the Kubler–Ross model and Lazarus and Folkman's transactional model. It examines how individuals adapt coping mechanisms during the pandemic, emphasising the significance of problem-focused and emotion-focused strategies. It highlights the unique challenges faced during the COVID-19 pandemic, such as loss, isolation, and uncertainty. It explores how people turn to electronic media platforms like social media and online entertainment for support and distraction. Drawing on existing literature, the chapter underscores the importance of electronic media as a coping mechanism, acknowledging both positive and negative effects on mental health. It concludes by advocating for further research into media-based coping strategies and emphasises the potential of digital platforms for supporting resilience and well-being during times of crisis.

In conclusion, the impact of the COVID-19 pandemic extends far beyond the statistics and numbers, as evidenced by the poignant case study of the 18-year-old boy and his family. This crisis has unleashed a cascade of psycho-physiological events that have reshaped our understanding of normalcy and resilience. From the breakdown of healthcare systems to the emergence of social stigma, the pandemic has left indelible marks on societies and individuals worldwide. However, amidst the chaos and uncertainty, there have been glimpses of hope and resilience manifested in coping strategies ranging from spirituality to technological innovation. As researchers and psychologists, we must continue to document and understand the long-term effects of this crisis while also exploring avenues for effective intervention and support. By acknowledging the profound impact of COVID-19 on mental health and well-being, we can work towards building a more resilient and compassionate society in the aftermath of the pandemic. We can emerge stronger from this crisis through collaboration and perseverance, armed with the knowledge and understanding needed to confront future challenges with courage and resilience.

Acknowledgement

Editors express gratitude to all the contributors, peer reviewers, and our editorial manager Ms. Lucy for all the support throughout the project.

References

Channa, A., Popescu, N., Skibinska, J., & Burget, R. (2021). The rise of wearable devices during the COVID-19 pandemic: A systematic review. *Sensors (Basel, Switzerland), 21*(17), 5787. https://doi.org/10.3390/s21175787

Dunn, S. H., & Conley, Y. P. (2015). A systematic review of genetic influences on coping. *Biological Research for Nursing, 17*(1), 87–93. https://doi.org/10.1177/1099800414527340

Mehta, K., Mehta, S., Chalana, H., Singh, H., & Thaman, R. G. (2020). Effectiveness of Rajyoga meditation as an adjunct to first-line treatment in patients with obsessive-compulsive disorder. *Indian Journal of Psychiatry, 62*(6), 684–689. https://doi.org/10.4103/psychiatry.IndianJPsychiatry_401_19

MyGov.in. (2024). *Covid19 statewise status*. Retrieved 19 February 2024, from https://www.mygov.in/corona-data/covid19-statewise-status

Population of India. (n.d.). *India population 2024: StatisticsTimes.com*. Retrieved 19 February 2024, from https://statisticstimes.com/demographics/country/india-population.php

Seyed Alinaghi, S., Afsahi, A. M., Shahidi, R., Afzalian, A., Mirzapour, P., Eslami, M., Ahmadi, S., Matini, P., Yarmohammadi, S., Saeed, T, Z, S., Asili, P., Paranjkhoo, P., Ramezani, M., Nooralioghli, P. S., Sanaati, F., Amiri, F. I., Emamgholizade, B. E., Mansouri, S., Pashaei, A., Mehraeen, E., ... Hackett, D. (2023). Social stigma during COVID-19: A systematic review. *Sage Open Medicine, 11*, 20503121231208273. https://doi.org/10.1177/20503121231208273

Wadman, M., Couzin-Frankel, J., Kaiser, J., & Matacic, C. (2020). A rampage through the body. *Science (New York, N.Y.), 368*(6489), 356–360. https://doi.org/10.1126/science.368.6489.356

World Health Organization (WHO). (2023, August 9). *Coronavirus Disease (Covid-19)*. World Health Organization. https://www.who.int/news-room/fact-sheets/detail/coronavirus-disease-(covid-19)

Internet Source

Psychiatry.org – Stigma, Prejudice and Discrimination Against People with Mental Illness.

1 Psychosocial Consequences of COVID-19 across Age Groups

A Systematic Review

Anita Manglani, Navkiran Kalsi, Shubham Prasad, Shreyas Babel, Nudrat Jahan, and Megha Sharma

Introduction

The COVID-19 pandemic has had a far-reaching impact on societies worldwide, disrupting lives, economies, and healthcare systems. Social distancing and isolation measures, lockdowns, and closures of educational institutions and workplaces were implemented strictly to curb the virus' spread. However, many unintended effects of these measures have also been observed. The COVID-19 pandemic has had a profound and lasting impact on individuals of all age groups, but the challenges and vulnerabilities experienced by each are unique.

The impact of the pandemic can be traced to the various aspects of human life, including the psychosocial sphere. Psychosocial characteristics result from an individual's psychological development within social and cultural contexts. According to the American Psychological Association (2020), the "psychosocial" is an "intersection and interaction of social, cultural, and environmental influences on the mind and behaviour". The psychosocial perspective on human behaviour examines the relationship between these factors and how they shape their behaviour (Woodward, 2015).

Psychosocial characteristics can indeed be predictors of socialisation across the human developmental course, and the importance of this relationship may vary based on age. A vast body of clinical and non-clinical literature has focused on a wide range of the psychosocial impact of COVID-19; however, methodological constraints of research limit these findings from drawing an overall conclusion (De Risio et al., 2023; Gnanapragasam et al., 2022)

In this context, the present study is assumed to fill the gap by addressing the comprehensive consequences of COVID-19 with empirical evidence.

The present research article synthesises existing literature and integrates various perspectives to develop a comprehensive understanding of the psychosocial consequences of COVID-19. It seeks to identify common themes and trends in the psychosocial effects experienced by children, adolescents, adults, and older adults. These insights will help in identifying the vulnerabilities of each age group. Thus, this study aims to inform policymakers, healthcare professionals, and researchers about the specific needs and challenges that different age cohorts

DOI: 10.4324/9781003454984-2

face. This study can enable the comprehensive and inclusive development of interventions, support systems, and public health strategies that address the diverse needs of individuals.

Methods

Aim

To study the psychosocial consequences of COVID-19 across different age groups through systematic review.

Data Collection

This review study followed the guidelines described under the Preferred Reporting Items for Systematic Reviews and Meta-Analyses- PRISMA (Page et al., 2021). A systematic literature review was conducted to understand the psychosocial consequences of COVID-19 across different age groups. A comprehensive search was conducted using five research databases: Web of Science, Scopus, PubMed, Google Scholar, and UGC-listed journals published between 2020 and 2023. The studies were retrieved using the keywords "COVID-19", "Pandemic", "Psychosocial", "Psychological", and "Social", which were found relevant to screen the research related to psychosocial consequences of COVID-19 across different age groups.

The search strategy was executed under three phases: search, screening, and selection. The key terms used were "COVID-19", "Pandemic", "Psychosocial", and "Psychological" "Social". COVID-19-related articles with at least two of the proposed key terms were retrieved. Each potentially relevant article was sorted into age groups: Children, adolescents, adults, old age, and common age. The articles were then screened based on Population (P) –children, adolescents, adults, and old; Intervention (I) – COVID-19; Comparison (C) – None; and Outcome (O) –psychosocial consequences. It is also known as PICO criteria. Potentially relevant articles were further shortlisted for full-text analysis. Three researchers did the final selection of articles. Finally, articles were selected based on the consensus of at least two researchers mentioned as authors in the current review.

Study Selection Criteria

The inclusion criteria of the studies:

- Articles published in the English language.
- Studies on non-clinical populations.
- The age groups of the population were based on Erik Erikson's 8 Stages of Psychosocial Development, which were children aged 12 and below, adolescents

aged 13–18 years, adults aged 19–65 years, and old age above 65 years (Legg and Lewis, 2023).

The exclusion criteria of the studies were:

- Articles published in languages other than English.
- Qualitative studies.
- Studies do not provide specific information about the sample age groups.
- Studies on clinical population.

Risk of Bias

Two reviewers evaluated the risk of bias for selected articles. They independently rated the quality of included studies using the National Institutes of Health Quality Assessment Tool for Systematic Reviews and Meta-Analyses, 2021 (Table 1.1).

Data Analysis

A data summary analysis was conducted on the relevant data that was collected. We utilised a data summary analysis once the relevant studies had been collected. Two authors of this review independently extracted data on the psychosocial consequences of COVID-19, which were then organised into summary tables. Psychosocial impacts were analysed using NVivo-20, and its Word-Cloud feature summarised the findings (Figure 1.1).

Results

The literature search yielded 13,632 academic research articles through database search engines. In total, 7,322 duplicate articles were removed. After excluding the duplicates, 5,083 articles were screened based on title and PICO criteria. A total of 302 articles were found to be eligible for full-text reading. Among 302, 261 were excluded based on criteria, such as qualitative studies, clinical population, no consensus among reviewers, and not in English. Collectively, 41 articles were included in the present systematic review study. These definitive studies include 7 studies for children, 4 for adolescents, 27 for adults, and 3 for older age groups. Based on the findings from each study, the psychosocial impacts were summarised and analysed using NVivo-20. As a result, we obtained the Word Cloud as depicted in the respective age group in the result section. Psychosocial Impacts of COVID-19 identified across age groups are described as follows:

Children

Only 7 out of 41 studies were found to be relevant for the given age range of children. The two main psychosocial effects of COVID-19 were found to be anxiety in children and sleep patterns that were disturbed. Other psychosocial effects were decreased social engagement, fear, despair, and behavioural and emotional issues. The psychosocial impacts identified are depicted in Figure 1.2 and Table 1.2.

Table 1.1 Quality Ratings of Included Studies According to the NIH Quality Assessment of Systematic Reviews and Meta-Analyses Studies for Various Age Groups

Age Group	S.No.	First Author	1	2	3	4	5	6	7	8	9	10	11	12	13	14	R1	R2
								Question									*Overall Rating*	
Children	1	Alnamnakani	√	√	√	√	√	√	√	√	√	√	√	*	*	f	f
	2	Zainudeen	√	√	√	√	√	√	√	√	√	√	√	*	*	f	f
	3	Theuring	√	√	√	√	√	√	√	√	√	√	√	*	*	f	f
	4	Malhi	√	√	√	√	√	√	√	√	√	√	√	*	*	f	f
	5	McKune	√	√	√	√	√	√	√	√	√	√	√	*	*	f	f
	6	Khoory	√	√	√	√	√	√	√	√	√	√	√	*	*	f	f
	7	Yurteri	√	√	√	√	√	√	√	√	√	√	√	*	*	f	f
Adolescents	1	Von Soest	√	√	√	√	√	√	√	√	√	√	√	*	*	f	f
	2	Romm	√	√	√	√	√	√	√	√	√	√	√	*	*	f	f
	3	Michael L	v	√	√	√	√	√	√	√	√	√	√	*	*	f	f
	4	Dale	√	√	√	√	√	√	√	√	√	√	√	*	*	f	f
Adult	1	Smallwood	√	√	√	√	√	√	√	√	√	√	√	*	*	f	f
	2	Jerg-Bretzke	√	√	√	√	√	√	√	√	√	√	√	*	*	f	f
	3	Fteropoulli	√	√	√	√	√	√	√	√	√	√	√	*	*	f	f
	4	Romm	√	√	√	√	√	√	√	√	√	√	√	*	*	f	f
	5	Norman	√	√	√	√	√	√	√	√	√	√	√	*	*	f	f
	6	Lamb	√	√	√	√	√	√	√	√	√	√	√	*	*	f	f
	7	Kovner	√	√	√	√	√	√	√	√	√	√	√	*	*	f	f
	8	Kirk	√	√	√	√	√	√	√	√	√	√	√	*	*	f	f
	9	Reskati	√	√	√	√	√	√	√	√	√	√	√	*	*	f	f
	10	Ogrodniczuk	√	√	√	√	√	√	√	√	√	√	√	*	*	f	f
	11	Magro	√	√	√	√	√	√	√	√	√	√	√	*	*	f	f
	12	Kumar D	√	√	v	√	√	√	√	√	√	√	√	*	*	f	f
	13	Bezerra	√	√	√	√	√	√	√	√	√	√	√	*	*	f	f
	14	El-Monshed	√	√	√	√	√	√	√	√	√	√	√	*	*	f	f
	15	Uribe-Restrepo	√	√	√	√	√	√	√	√	√	√	√	*	*	f	f
	16	Ramalho	√	√	√	√	√	√	√	√	√	√	√	*	*	f	f
	17	Munoz-Munoz	√	√	v	√	√	√	√	√	√	√	√	*	*	f	f
	18	Rothman	√	√	√	√	√	√	√	√	√	√	√	*	*	f	f
	19	Cam	√	√	√	√	√	√	√	√	√	√	√	*	*	f	f
	20	Siow	√	√	√	√	√	√	√	√	√	√	√	*	*	f	f
	21	Umeizudike	√	√	√	√	√	√	√	√	√	√	√	*	*	f	f
	22	Mato	√	√	√	√	√	√	√	√	√	√	√	*	*	f	f
	23	Ijah	√	√	√	√	√	√	√	√	√	√	√	*	*	f	f
	24	Frank	√	√	√	√	√	√	√	√	√	√	√	*	*	f	f
	25	Duan	√	√	√	√	√	√	√	√	√	√	√	*	*	f	f
	26	Li	√	√	√	√	√	√	√	√	√	√	√	*	*	f	f
	27	Sagherian	√	√	√	√	√	√	√	√	√	√	√	*	*	f	f

(*Continued*)

Table 1.1 (Continued)

Age Group	S.No.	First Author	1	2	3	4	5	6	7	8	9	10	11	12	13	14	R1	R2
														Question				*Overall Rating*	
Older	1	Hansen	√	√	√	√	√	√	√	√	√	√	√	√	*	*	f	f
	2	Galea	√	√	√	√	√	√	√	√	√	√	√	√	*	*	f	f
	3	Saha	√	√	√	√	√	√	√	√	√	√	√	√	*	*	f	f

Note: NIH, National Institutes of Health; √, Yes; NR, not reported; *, cannot determine; NA, not applicable; R, Reviewer; f, fair.

The NIH Quality Assessment for Observational Cohort and Cross-Sectional Studies poses eight questions [14]: 1. Was this paper's research question or objective clearly stated? 2. Was the study population specified and defined? 3. Was the participation rate of eligible persons at least 50%? 4. Were all the subjects selected or recruited from the same or similar populations (including the same time)? Were inclusion and exclusion criteria for being in the study prespecified and applied uniformly to all participants? 5. Was a sample size justification, power description, or variance and effect estimates provided? 6. For the analyses in this paper, were the exposure(s) of interest measured before the outcome(s) being measured? 7. Was the timeframe sufficient to reasonably expect to see an association between exposure and outcome if it existed? 8. For exposures that can vary in amount or level, did the study examine different levels of the exposure as related to the outcome (e.g., categories of exposure or exposure measured as a continuous variable)? 9. Were the exposure measures (independent variables) clearly defined, valid, reliable, and implemented consistently across all study participants? 10. Was the exposure(s) assessed more than once over time? 11. Were the outcome measures (dependent variables) clearly defined, valid, reliable, and implemented consistently across all study participants? 12. Were the outcome assessors blinded to the exposure status of participants? 13. Was loss to follow-up after baseline 20% or less? 14. Were key potential confounding variables measured and adjusted statistically for their impact on the relationship between exposure(s) and outcome(s)?

Adolescents

After going through 41 studies, only 4 studies were identified for the adolescent's age group. The major psychosocial impacts of COVID-19 were identified as depression and anxiety in adolescents. In addition to these aforementioned impacts, the other explored suicidal ideation stress. The psychosocial impacts identified are depicted in Figure 1.3 and Table 1.3.

Adult

Among 41 studies, 27 studies were recognised for the Adult age group. The major psychosocial impacts of COVID-19 were identified as anxiety, depression, stress, and post-traumatic stress disorder (PTSD) in adults. Apart from these aforementioned impacts, the others were disclosed as worry, psychological distress, alcohol use, fear, poor quality of life, common mental disorders, alcohol use, physical and emotional exhaustion, and so on. The psychosocial impacts identified are depicted in Figure 1.4 and Table 1.4.

Older

After going through 41 studies, only 3 studies were identified for the old age group. The major psychosocial impacts of COVID-19 were identified as social isolation in

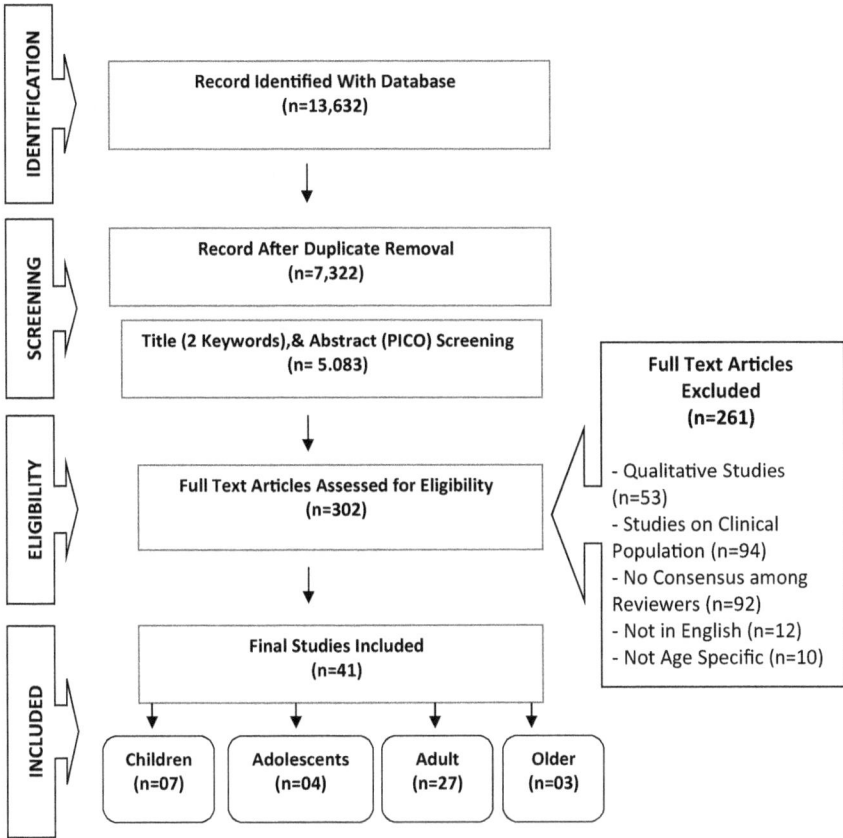

IDENTIFICATION

SCREENING

ELIGIBILITY

INCLUDED

Record Identified With Database
(n=13,632)

Record After Duplicate Removal
(n=7,322)

Title (2 Keywords),& Abstract (PICO) Screening
(n= 5.083)

Full Text Articles Assessed for Eligibility
(n=302)

Full Text Articles
Excluded
(n=261)

- Qualitative Studies
(n=53)
- Studies on Clinical
Population (n=94)
- No Consensus among
Reviewers (n=92)
- Not in English (n=12)
- Not Age Specific (n=10)

Final Studies Included
(n=41)

Children
(n=07)

Adolescents
(n=04)

Adult
(n=27)

Older
(n=03)

Figure 1.1 PRISMA Flow Diagram Depicting the Selection Process.

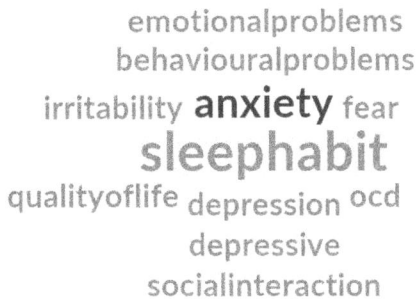

emotionalproblems
behaviouralproblems
irritability **anxiety** fear
sleephabit
qualityoflife depression ocd
depressive
socialinteraction

Figure 1.2 Word Cloud for Children.

Table 1.2 Studies Highlighted the Psychosocial Impact on Children

S.No.	First Author (Year)	Psychosocial Impact	Key Findings
1	Alnamnakani et al. (2022)	Anxiety Depression	28.1% of children had elevated anxiety levels. 4.4% of children had severe depression.
3	Theuring (2022)	Anxiety Fear Social interaction	Anxiety symptoms increased. Fear of infection increased. Social interaction was reduced.
4	Khoory (2022)	Irritability	In children, parental fluctuating moods were correlated with high irritability (74%).
5	Malhi (2021)	· Emotional problems · Behavioural problems	Emotional and behavioural problems of children were in the abnormal range
6	McKune (2021)	· Anxiety · Depressive · OCD	Increased risk for depressive symptoms, anxiety-related symptoms, and OCD-related symptoms were associated with loss of household income. The risk for depressive, anxiety, and OCD symptoms was found to be significantly higher in females. Parental practices to fight the coronavirus were linked to a significant increase in depression in children. In children, a rise in anxiety and obsessive-compulsive symptoms were associated with lower school levels.
7	Yurteri (2021)	· Bedtime · Resistance · Delayed sleep onset · Night awakenings · Parasomnia · Daytime sleep · Sleep problems · Anxiety · Depression · Quality of life	· Increased bedtime resistance · Delayed sleep onset · Increased night awakening · Increased parasomnias · Daytime sleepiness · Increased anxiety · Increased depression · Reduced quality of life

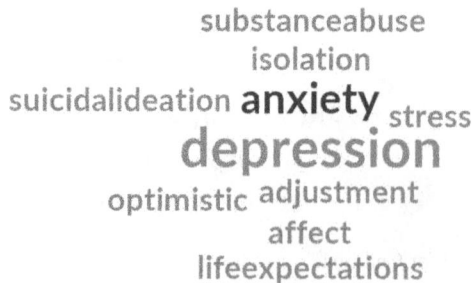

Figure 1.3 Word Cloud for Adolescence.

Table 1.3 Studies Highlighted the Psychosocial Impact on Adolescence

S.No.	First Author (Year)	Psychosocial Impact	Key Findings
1	Von Soest (2022)	Depression Less optimistic Substance abuse	Increase in symptoms of depression Less optimistic for future life expectations Decrease in use of cannabis and alcohol
2	Dale (2022)	Depression Suicidal ideation	Females reported a decline in mental health (i.e., well-being, depression, insomnia, suicidal ideation) Among boys, an increase in suicidal thoughts was seen
3	Romm (2021a,b)	Depression Affect Isolation Adjustment	Increases in depressive symptoms Negative affect has reportedly increased; Positive affect has reportedly decreased Increase in social isolation Negative changes in adolescent adjustment
4	Tee (2020)	Anxiety Stress Depression	Moderate-to-severe anxiety levels Psychological impacts were reported moderate to severe Symptoms related to depression appeared to range between moderate to severe

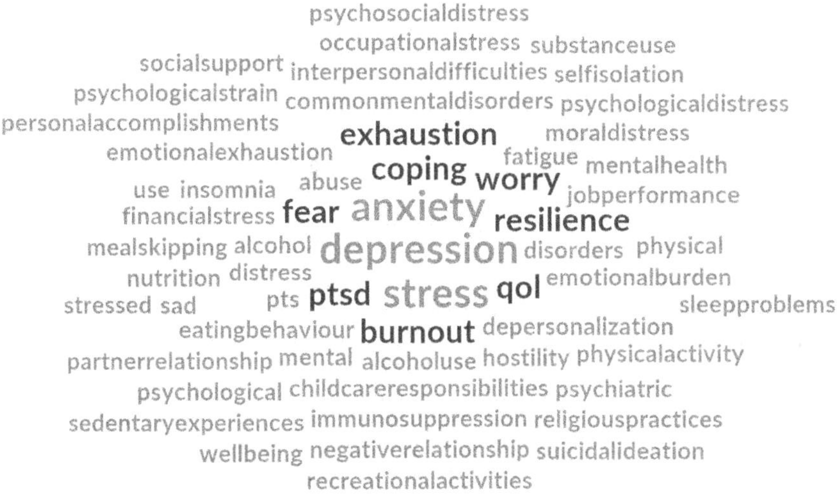

psychosocialdistress
occupationalstress substanceuse
socialsupport interpersonaldifficulties selfisolation
psychologicalstrain commonmentaldisorders psychologicaldistress
personalaccomplishments **exhaustion** moraldistress
emotionalexhaustion fatigue mentalhealth
use insomnia abuse **coping worry** jobperformance
financialstress **fear anxiety** resilience
mealskipping alcohol **depression** disorders physical
nutrition distress emotionalburden
stressed sad pts **ptsd stress qol** sleepproblems
eatingbehaviour **burnout** depersonalization
partnerrelationship mental alcoholuse hostility physicalactivity
psychological childcareresponsibilities psychiatric
sedentaryexperiences immunosuppression religiouspractices
wellbeing negativerelationship suicidalideation
recreationalactivities

Figure 1.4 Word Cloud for Adult.

Table 1.4 Studies Highlighted the Psychosocial Impact on Adult

S.No.	First Author (Year)	Psychosocial Impact	Key Findings
1	Magro (2022)	Depression	Elevated levels of depression
		Anxiety	Elevated levels of burnout
		Burnout	Elevated levels of Stress
		Stress	Elevated levels of anxiety
		Quality of life	Low levels of quality of life
		Resilience	Moderate levels of resilience
2	El-Monshed (2022)	Depression	Depression reported by 74.5% students
		Anxiety	Anxiety reported by 47.1% students
		Stress	Stress reported by 40.5% students
		Coping	More involved in problem-solving coping strategies, such as planning and taking action
			Less use of maladaptive coping strategies, such as expressing emotions, avoiding the problem, and substance use
3	Uribe-Restrepo (2022)	Anxiety	Mild to moderate anxiety symptoms by 29%; moderate-severe 18%, and severe anxiety by 6.0% of the population. Symptoms of anxiety were linked to financial insecurity, specifically the
		Depression	inability to afford food.
			Females documented higher depressive symptoms
4	Ramalho (2022)		During lockdown the surveyed sample reported:
		•Meal skipping	•Skipping meals
		•Eating behaviour	•Overeating
			•Grazing eating behaviour
			•Loss of control over eating
			•Binge eating episodes
5	Muñoz-Muñoz (2022)		Intensive Care Units (ICU) nurses reported:
		Sleep problems	•Problems with sleep
		Anxiety	•Anxiety
		Stress	•Stress
		Job performance	•Worsening work performance
6	Rothmann (2022)		COVID-19 was associated with symptoms of:
		Depression	Depression
		Anxiety	Anxiety
		Stress	Stress
7	Cam (2022)		University students reported symptoms of
		Depression	Depression
		Anxiety	Anxiety
		Stress	Stress
		PTSD	PTSD
		Emotional Burden	Emotional Burden

(*Continued*)

Table 1.4 (Continued)

S.No.	First Author (Year)	Psychosocial Impact	Key Findings
8	Siow (2022)	Psychosocial Distress	Health care workers are at risk of psychosocial distress
9	Umeizudike (2022)	Worry	Majority of students were•worried about contracting COVID-19
10	Mato (2022)	Stress •Psychological distress	Highly Stressed Experienced severe psychological distress
11	Ijah (2022)	Well-Being	Poor well-being index among 31.6% of respondents, 17.1% reported a Fair well-being index, 19.7% reported good well-being index, and •31.6% reported excellent well-being index
12	Frank (2022)	Depression Anxiety	Half of the medical students reported feeling depressed 62% reported high anxiety levels
13	Smallwood (2021)	Anxiety Burnout Depression Resilience	Anxiety symptoms ranged between mild to severe Burnout ranged from Moderate to Severe Symptoms of depression ranged from mild to severe High resilience
14	Jerg-Bretzke (2021)	Occupational stress Fear Physical exhaustion Mental exhaustion Defective coping	Increase in stress during the pandemic. Highest fear of infecting others Extreme mental and physical exhaustion People living alone utilised more defective strategies of coping.
15	Theodora Fteropoulli (2021)	Anxiety Depression Quality of life	The prevalence of anxiety ranging between moderate to severe was 27.6% The prevalence of depression was 26.8% Occupational burnout and depression were major contributors to inadequate quality of life during COVID-19.
16	Romm (2021a,b)	Childcare responsibilities Resilience Negative relationship Alcohol use Physical activity Sedentary experiences Poor Nutrition Depression	Negative mental health impacts are more correlated with increased childcare responsibilities. Negative mental health impacts are more correlated with lower resilience. People in relationships experienced negative relationship impacts Increased alcohol use Decreased physical activity More sedentary lifestyle Poorer nutrition Depressive symptoms predicted more negative mental health impacts

(Continued)

Table 1.4 (Continued)

S.No.	First Author (Year)	Psychosocial Impact	Key Findings
17	Norman (2021)	Moral Distress	The majority of the sample experienced moral distress.
		PTSD	Moral distress is significantly related to severity and COVID-19-related PTSD symptoms.
		Burnout Interpersonal difficulties	Moral distress is also associated with burnout, and work and interpersonal difficulties
18	Lamb (2021)	Common mental disorders	High likelihood of prevalent mental health conditions (CMDs)
		PTSD	Substantial levels of PTSD
		Anxiety	Declining levels of anxiety
		Depression	Lower levels of depression
		Alcohol use	Higher alcohol misuse
19	Kovner (2021)	Depression	Higher depression
		Anxiety	Higher anxiety
20	Kirk (2021)	Depression	Depressive symptoms in 39.1% respondents
		Anxiety	Anxiety was seen in 47.7% respondents
		Stress	Stress was seen in 24.7% respondents
21	Kumar (2021)	Depression	Depression ranging from moderate to severe
		Anxiety	Anxiety reaching moderate to serious levels of severity
		Stress	Moderate to critical levels of stress
22	Ogrodniczuk (2021)	Mental health	Negative impacts on Mental health
		Financial stress	Moderate financial stress (50% sample)
		Partner relationship •Suicidal ideation	Harmful effect on their connection with their romantic partner.
		Abuse	Suicidal ideation (42.2% sample)
			30.9% engages in some kind of abuse
23	Reskati (2021)	Depression	Moderate-to-severe levels of depression
		Anxiety	Anxiety ranging from moderate to severe
		Stress	Stress reaching moderate to severe levels
		PTSD	Possible PTSD
		Immuno-suppression	Immuno-suppression
24	Duan (2020)	Fear	The level of fear significantly decreased over time
		Depression	The severity of depression significantly increased over time. Factors that may predict the likelihood of depression include being of a younger age, experiencing a higher level of perceived stress, having a lower income, and undergoing quarantine.
		Hostility	Hostility predictor: Younger age, increased perceived stress and low-income
		Coping	Negative coping strategy associated with rise in hostility
		Social support	The presence of social support acts as a buffer against feelings of hostility.

(*Continued*)

Table 1.4 (Continued)

S.No.	First Author (Year)	Psychosocial Impact	Key Findings
25	Bezerra (2020)	Worry about self-isolation	Worry about Adapt to new reality
			Changed routine after self-isolation
		Sad	Experiencing the feeling of sadness and anxiety
		Religious practices, Recreational activities	High engaging in physical activity, spiritual practices, and/or leisure activities
26	Li (2020)	PTSD	Age, occupation, education level, and Psychiatric disorders are significantly correlated with a high level of PTSD
		Coping	Problem-focused coping was significantly associated with high levels of PTSD
			Emotional and problem-solving coping strategies were found to be more effective for individuals with better psychiatric status
27	Sagherian (2020)	Insomnia	Sub-threshold insomnia
		Fatigue	Moderate to high levels of chronic fatigue, high acute fatigue
		Emotional exhaustion	Increased emotional exhaustion
		Depersonalisation	Increased depersonalisation
		PTS	High post-traumatic stress (PTS)
		Psychological distress	Moderate psychological distress
		Personal accomplishments	Increased personal accomplishments

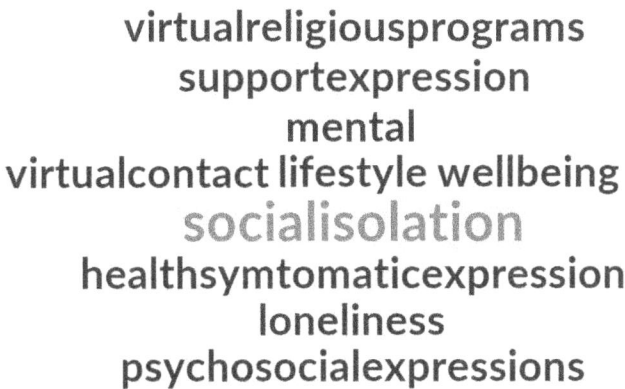

Figure 1.5 Word Cloud for Older.

Table 1.5 Studies Highlighted the Psychosocial Impact for Older

S.No.	First Author (Year)	Psychosocial Impact	Key Findings
1	Hansen (2022)	Loneliness Well-being	Individuals who are women, single, and older are more likely to be affected by loneliness disproportionately Broad, substantial declines in psychosocial well-being
2	Galea (2022)	Lifestyle Virtual contact with family Friends declined over time Virtual religious programs Social isolation	Healthy lifestyle maintained The frequency of virtual contact with family and friends decreased over time Religious programs conducted virtually. Increase in social isolation
3	Saha (2020)	Psychosocial expressions Mental health expression Support expression	Psychosocial expressions significantly increased Increased mental health symptomatic expression Increased support expression

old age. Moreover, the other impacts were identified as loneliness, virtual contacts, and so on. The psychosocial impacts identified are depicted in Figure 1.5 and Table 1.5.

Discussion

The COVID-19 pandemic has had widespread and significant psychosocial impacts across different age groups. This review identified key findings regarding the psychosocial consequences experienced by children, adolescents, adults, and the elderly.

The review consistently identified anxiety and depression as the most common psychosocial impact of the pandemic across all age groups. The COVID-19 pandemic caused individuals to be anxious. Children, adolescents, and adults experienced an increase in their level of anxiety (Tee et al., 2020; Yurteri & Sarigedik, 2021; Dale et al., 2022; El-Monshed et al., 2022; Dale et al., 2022). Not only healthcare professionals, despite being highly resilient (Smallwood et al., 2021; Rothmann et al., 2022), but also students (El-Monshed et al., 2022) and parents (Yurteri & Sarigedik, 2021) felt more anxious than the pre-pandemic period.

Children, adolescents, and adults alike suffered from depression during the pandemic. For children, increased depression and anxiety levels resulted in increased sleep problems (Yurteri & Sarigedik, 2021; Zainudeen et al., 2021; Alnamnakani et al., 2022). Meanwhile, adolescents experienced increased depression (Von Soest et al., 2022) as during the pandemic, they felt isolated, confined in their homes away from their friends and support systems for long periods. Depression was also found in the adult population as well in the range of mild to severe (Reskati et al., 2021; Kirk et al., 2021; Magro et al., 2022; Lamb et al., 2021; Kovner et al., 2021; Fteropoulli et al., 2021, Cam et al., 2022; Kumar et al., 2021; Von Soest et al., 2022). Frontline healthcare workers were the ones to bear the brunt of it, with a majority reporting symptoms of depression (Smallwood et al., 2021; Uribe-Restrepo et al., 2022; Rothmann et al., 2022). Students did not fare much better, as indicated by the findings of El-Monshed et al. (2022), Duan et al. (2020), and Cam et al. (2022).

Children have been affected by disruptions in their daily routines, leading to sleep problems, emotional and behavioural issues, and fear of contracting COVID-19. Emotional and behavioural problems in children have been linked to parental stress and their negative and positive affect (Malhi et al., 2021; Khoory et al., 2022). Sleep problems (Yurteri & Sarigedik, 2021), OCD-related symptoms (McKune et al., 2021), and anxiety and fear of COVID-19 have resulted in detriments in the health-related quality of life of children (Theuring et al., 2022).

Adolescents have experienced a significant increase in depression, anxiety, and stress during the pandemic. Positive emotional experiences and optimism have decreased, while negative emotional experiences and feelings of isolation increased (Romm et al., 2021a,b; Von Soest et al., 2022). Increased screen time and limited social interactions have contributed to these impacts. Girls, younger adolescents, groups with a low socio-economic position and other such vulnerable groups experienced more drastic impacts. A significant percentage of adolescents, regardless of gender difference, reported having suicidal ideation, resulting in deterioration in mental health (Dale et al., 2022).

Adults have been heavily impacted by the pandemic, experiencing anxiety, depression, stress, PTSD, burnout, distress, sleep problems, and fear. Various factors, such as being female, working as frontline healthcare staff, and having a relative or acquaintance affected by COVID-19, have contributed to higher anxiety levels. Frontline healthcare workers, including physicians, nurses, and midwives, have reported higher levels of depression (Rothmann et al., 2022). Stress was common during the pandemic, with most people experiencing an increase since the first wave (Jerg-Bretzke et al., 2021; Muñoz-Muñoz et al., 2022). Dysfunctional coping strategies exacerbated negative psychological and psychiatric problems (Li, 2020; Jerg-Bretzke et al., 2021; Fteropoulli et al., 2021) and increased hostility (Duan et al., 2020). PTSD, burnout, and moral distress have been observed among healthcare workers. Alcohol use and quality of life have also been affected by the pandemic. University students also showed substantial symptoms of stress and worried about academic loss (El-Monshed et al., 2022). Healthcare workers faced the worst of the pandemic at the frontlines and suffered from burnout (Smallwood et al., 2021; Magro et al., 2022) and PTSD (Reskati et al., 2021; Lamb et al., 2021; Cam et al., 2022) too. Resilience was found to be in an inverse relationship with negative psychosocial impacts of the pandemic by the studies by Romm et al. (2021a,b) and Magro et al. (2022). Apart from those mentioned above, other consequences were abuse, emotional exhaustion, hostility, interpersonal difficulties, physical activity, self-isolation, sleep problems, post-traumatic growth, and so on.

The elderly population has faced social isolation, lifestyle changes, loneliness, mental health concerns, and challenges in psychosocial and support expression. They have been more vulnerable to contracting the virus and have experienced drastic changes in their social circles and lifestyles. Virtual contact and religious programs have helped maintain connections, but the impacts have been disproportionately borne by women, single individuals, and older adults. Additionally, a study by Saha et al. (2020) noted that negative mental health outcomes (anxiety, depression, stress, and suicidal ideation) and their support expressed for well-being (emotional and informational support) significantly increased during the COVID-19 for elderly people. In the data collected, the negative Psychosocial outcomes for this age group also included loneliness psychological ill-being (worried, anxious, depressed) (Hansen et al., 2022). However, a healthy lifestyle was maintained among most of the elderly. Moreover, virtual contact with family and friends declined over time, virtual religious programs were maintained, and social isolation increased (Galea et al., 2022).

Overall, the psychosocial impacts of the COVID-19 pandemic have been extensive and have affected individuals of all age groups. Anxiety and depression have consistently emerged as the most common consequences across all age groups. Factors such as gender, occupation (especially healthcare workers), and personal circumstances have influenced the severity and nature of the impacts. It is crucial to address these psychosocial consequences and provide support to individuals to mitigate the chronic consequences on mental well-being.

Limitations and Strengths of the Study

This systematic review of literature addresses the psychosocial impact of the COVID-19 pandemic on individuals of all age groups from all over the world. However, there are certain limitations of the present study. First, only English language research literature was included. This may have led to the exclusion of a considerable body of non-English studies relevant to the present review. Second, this review does not include the grey literature database. As a result, some important points of interest may have been left out. Also, there is a possibility that certain cultural factors were not highlighted. Thus, generalising the findings of this review may not be appropriate in all contexts.

Still, despite these limitations, the present study may boast several strengths. First, this study presents a systematic review of all the available material on the psychosocial impact of the COVID-19 pandemic across all age groups. It addresses the research on all age groups, including children, teenagers, adults, and senior citizens. Second, this review is not limited to a geographic location or occupation. Studies from countries all over the globe have been included – USA, Egypt, Italy, Pakistan, Australia, Bangladesh, and so on. People in different occupations are also included – from teachers and students to healthcare workers working in different positions in the system, to parents and others. Thus, this comprehensive review covers the impact faced by individuals from all over the world and may be utilised to help develop a better grasp of the pandemic's psychosocial impact.

Conclusion

To conclude, the present systematic review reveals depression, anxiety, stress, fear, sleep problems, and feelings of loneliness and isolation to be prevalent in populations of all ages as a cause for concern. The strength of the study reflected that it covers various countries all over the world. This serves as evidence of the negative outcomes of the COVID-19 pandemic. From little children to elderly people above the age of 60, the pandemic has left no human being untouched. To cope with the change the pandemic brought and its negative impacts, the world needs to work together. The need is to develop targeted interventions, support systems, and public health strategies for different age groups. Those in positions of authority and power must use the resources and facilities available to them to help mitigate the pandemic's negative impacts and prepare for the long run by developing mental health safety nets.

These findings could contribute to developing targeted interventions, support systems, and public health strategies for different age groups. Insights on the psychosocial impacts of the pandemic gained through this review and the studies included herein underscore the need for the world to pay special heed to this particular sphere of human life. The findings of this review may help develop a better grasp of the consequences of the pandemic. It addresses research on all age groups from all over the world and is, therefore, a comprehensive work.

Author Contributions

Conceptualisation: Manglani, Kalsi and Babel; Methods: Manglani and Kalsi; Data Collection: Manglani, Kalsi, Sharma, Prasad, and Babel; Data analysis: Manglani and Kalsi; Writing: Manglani, Kalsi, Sharma, Jahan, and Prasad; Writing – review and editing: Manglani, Kalsi, and Jahan. All authors have read and agreed to the published version of the manuscript.

Acknowledgement

We are grateful to researchers whose studies provided invaluable data for this review.

References

Alnamnakani, M., Alenezi, S., Temsah, H., Alothman, M., Murshid, R. E., Alonazy, H., & Alqurashi, H. (2022). Psychosocial impact of lockdown on children due to COVID-19: A cross-sectional study. *Clinical Practice and Epidemiology in Mental Health, 18*(1). https://doi.org/10.2174/17450179-v18-e2203210

American Psychological Association. (2020). Psychosocial. In *APA dictionary of psychology*. https://dictionary.apa.org/psychosocial

Bezerra, C. B., Saintrain, M. V. D. L., Braga, D. R. A., Santos, F. D. S., Lima, A. O. P., Brito, E. H. S. D., & Pontes, C. D. B. (2020). Impacto psicossocial do isolamento durante pandemia de COVID-19 na população brasileira: análise transversal preliminar. *Saúde e Sociedade, 29*, e200412. https://doi.org/10.1590/S0104-12902020200412

Cam, H. H., Ustuner Top, F., & Kuzlu Ayyildiz, T. (2022). Impact of the COVID-19 pandemic on mental health and health-related quality of life among university students in Turkey. *Current Psychology, 41*(2), 1033–1042. https://doi.org/10.1007/s12144-021-01674-y

Dale, R., Jesser, A., Pieh, C., O'Rourke, T., Probst, T., & Humer, E. (2022). Mental health burden of high school students, and suggestions for psychosocial support, 1.5 years into the COVID-19 pandemic in Austria. *European Child & Adolescent Psychiatry*, 1–10. https://doi.org/10.1007/s00787-022-02032-4

De Risio, L., Pettorruso, M., Collevecchio, R., Collacchi, B., Boffa, M., Santorelli, M., et al. (2023). Staying connected: An umbrella review of meta-analyses on the push-and-pull of social connection in depression. *Journal of Affective Disorders.* https://doi.org/10.1016/j.jad.2023.10.112

Duan, H., Yan, L., Ding, X., Gan, Y., Kohn, N., & Wu, J. (2020). Impact of the COVID-19 pandemic on mental health in the general Chinese population: Changes, predictors and psychosocial correlates. *Psychiatry Research, 293*, 113396. https://doi.org/10.1016/j.psychres.2020.113396

El-Monshed, A. H., El-Adl, A. A., Ali, A. S., & Loutfy, A. (2022). University students under lockdown, the psychosocial effects and coping strategies during COVID-19 pandemic: A cross-sectional study in Egypt. *Journal of American College Health, 70*(3), 679–690. https://doi.org/10.1080/07448481.2021.1891086

Fteropoulli, T., Kalavana, T. V., Yiallourou, A., Karaiskakis, M., Koliou Mazeri, M., Vryonides, S., et al. (2021). Beyond the physical risk: Psychosocial impact and coping in healthcare professionals during the COVID-19 pandemic. *Journal of Clinical Nursing.* https://doi.org/10.1111/jocn.15938

Frank, V., Doshi, A., Demirjian, N. L., Fields, B. K., Song, C., Lei, X., et al. (2022). Educational, psychosocial, and clinical impact of SARS-CoV-2 (COVID-19) pandemic on medical students in the United States. *World Journal of Virology, 11*(3), 150. https://doi.org/10.5501/wjv.v11.i3.150

Galea, M., Sammut, A., Grech, P., Scerri, J., Calleja Bitar, D., & Dimech Sant, S. (2022). Psychosocial impact of COVID-19 on Malta's elderly. *Athens Journal of Health & Medical Sciences, 9*(1), 11–22. https://doi.org/10.30958/ajhms_v9i1.

Gnanapragasam, S. N., Hodson, A., Smith, L. E., Greenberg, N., Rubin, G. J., & Wessely, S. (2022). COVID-19 survey burden for health care workers: Literature review and audit. *Public Health, 206*, 94–101. https://doi.org/10.1016/j.puhe.2021.05.006

Hansen, T., Sevenius Nilsen, T., Knapstad, M., Skirbekk, V., Skogen, J., Vedaa, Ø, et al. (2022). Covid-fatigued? A longitudinal study of Norwegian older adults' psychosocial well-being before and during early and later stages of the COVID-19 pandemic. *European Journal of Ageing, 19*, 463–473. https://doi.org/10.1007/s10433-021-00648-0

Ijah, R. F. O. A., Onodingene, N., & Alabi, A. (2022). Clinical students in COVID-19 disease era: Knowledge & psychosocial impact. *Clinical Case Reports Open Access, 5*(1), 203. https://doi.org/10.46527/2582-5038.203

Jerg-Bretzke, L., Kempf, M., Jarczok, M. N., Weimer, K., Hirning, C., Gündel, H., et al. (2021). Psychosocial impact of the COVID-19 pandemic on healthcare workers and initial areas of action for intervention and prevention– the egePan/VOICE study. *International Journal of Environmental Research and Public Health, 18*(19), 10531. https://doi.org/10.3390/ijerph181910531

Khoory, B. J., Keuning, M. W., Fledderus, A. C., Cicchelli, R., Fanos, V., Khoory, J., et al. (2022). Psychosocial impact of 8 weeks COVID-19 quarantine on Italian parents and their children. *Matern Child Health Journal, 26*, 1312–1321. https://doi.org/10.1007/s10995-021-03311-3

Kirk, A. H., Chong, S. L., Kam, K. Q., Huang, W., Ang, L. S., Lee, J. H., et al. (2021). Psychosocial impact of the COVID-19 pandemic on paediatric healthcare workers. *Annals of the Academy of Medicine of Singapore, 50*(3), 203–211. https://doi.org/10.47102/annals-acadmedsg.2020527

Kovner, C., Raveis, V. H., Van Devanter, N., Yu, G., Glassman, K., & Ridge, L. J. (2021). The psychosocial impact on frontline nurses of caring for patients with COVID-19 during the first wave of the pandemic in New York City. *Nursing Outlook, 69*(5), 744–754. https://doi.org/10.1016/j.outlook.2021.03.019

Kumar, D., Saghir, T., Ali, G., Yasin, U., Furnaz, S., Karim, M., et al. (2021). Psychosocial impact of COVID-19 on healthcare workers at a Tertiary Care Cardiac Center of Karachi, Pakistan. *Journal of Occupational and Environmental Medicine, 63*(2), e59–e62. https://doi.org/10.1097/JOM.0000000000002094

Lamb, D., Gnanapragasam, S., Greenberg, N., Bhundia, R., Carr, E., Hotopf, M., et al. (2021). Psychosocial impact of the COVID-19 pandemic on 4378 UK healthcare workers and ancillary staff: Initial baseline data from a cohort study collected during the first wave of the pandemic. *Occupational and Environmental Medicine, 78*(11), 801–808. https://oem.bmj.com/content/78/11/801.abstract

Legg, T. J., & Lewis, R. (2023). *Erikson's 8 stages of psychosocial development, explained for parents.* Retrieved from https://www.healthline.com/health/parenting/erikson-stages#2-independence

Li, Q. (2020). Psychosocial and coping responses toward 2019 coronavirus diseases (COVID-19): A cross-sectional study within the Chinese general population. *QJM: An International Journal of Medicine, 113*(10), 731–738. https://doi.org/10.1093/qjmed/hcaa226

Magro, A., Gutiérrez-García, A., González-Álvarez, M., & Del Líbano, M. (2022). Psychosocial impact of the COVID-19 pandemic on healthcare professionals in Spain. *Sustainability, 14*(22), 15171. https://doi.org/10.3390/su142215171

Malhi, P., Bharti, B., & Sidhu, M. (2021) Stress and parenting during the COVID-19 pandemic: Psychosocial impact on children. *Indian Journal of Pediatrics, 88*, 481. https://doi.org/10.1007/s12098-021-03665-0

Mato, C. N., Ijah, R. F. O. A., Onodingene, N. M., Aaron, F. E., Owhonda, G., & Ogamba, M. I. (2022). Psychosocial impact of COVID-19 tests and positive results on clinical students screened during the second wave of COVID-19 pandemic in Rivers State, Nigeria. https://doi.org/10.9734/IJTDH/2022/v43i530591

McKune, S. L., Acosta, D., Diaz, N., Brittain, K., Joyce-Beaulieu, D., Maurelli, A. T., et al. (2021). Psychosocial health of school-aged children during the initial COVID-19 safer-at-home school mandates in Florida: A cross-sectional study. *BMC Public Health, 21*, 603. https://doi.org/10.1186/s12889-021-10540-2

Muñoz-Muñoz, M., Carretero-Bravo, J., Pérez-Muñoz, C., & Díaz-Rodríguez, M. (2022). Analysis of the psychosocial impact of the COVID-19 pandemic on the nursing staff of the intensive care units (ICU) in Spain. *In Healthcare, 10*(5), 796. https://doi.org/10.3390/healthcare10050796

National Institutes of Health Quality Assessment Tool for Systematic Reviews and Meta-Analyses. (2021). Retrieved from https://www.nhlbi.nih.gov/health-topics/study-quality-assessment-tools.

Norman, S. B., Feingold, J. H., Kaye-Kauderer, H., Kaplan, C. A., Hurtado, A., Kachadourian, L., et al. (2021). Moral distress in frontline healthcare workers in the initial epicentre of the COVID-19 pandemic in the United States: Relationship to PTSD symptoms, burnout, and psychosocial functioning. *Depression and Anxiety, 38*(10), 1007–1017. https://doi.org/10.1002/da.23205

NVivo qualitative data analysis. Version 20.2 [software]. Available from: QSR NVivo 20.2 Download (Free trial) – NVivo.exe (informer.com).

Ogrodniczuk, J. S., Rice, S. M., Kealy, D., Seidler, Z. E., Delara, M., & Oliffe, J. L. (2021). Psychosocial impact of the COVID-19 pandemic: A cross-sectional study of online help-seeking Canadian men. *Postgraduate Medicine, 133*(7), 750–759. https://doi.org/10.1080/00325481.2021.1873027

Page, M. J., McKenzie, J. E., Bossuyt, P. M., Boutron, I., Hoffmann, T. C., Mulrow, C. D., et al. (2021). The PRISMA 2020 statement: An updated guideline for reporting systematic reviews. *BMJ, 372*(n71). https://doi.org/10.1136/bmj.n71

Ramalho, S. M., Trovisqueira, A., de Lourdes, M., Gonçalves, S., Ribeiro, I., Vaz, A. R., et al. (2022). The impact of COVID-19 lockdown on disordered eating behaviours: The mediation role of psychological distress. *Eating and Weight Disorders-Studies on Anorexia, Bulimia and Obesity, 27*(1), 179–188. https://link.springer.com/article/10.1007/s40519-021-01128-1

Reskati, M. H., Shafizad, M., Aarabi, M., Hedayatizadeh-Omran, A., Khosravi, S., & Elyasi, F. (2021). Mental health status and psychosocial issues during Nationwide COVID-19 quarantine in Iran in 2020: A cross-sectional study in Mazandaran Province. *Current Psychology.* https://doi.org/10.1007/s12144-021-02011-z

Romm, K. F., Park, Y. W., Hughes, J. L., & Gentzler, A. L. (2021a). Risk and protective factors for changes in adolescent psychosocial adjustment during COVID-19. *Journal of Research on Adolescence, 31*(3), 546–559. https://doi.org/10.1111/jora.12667

Romm, K. F., Patterson, B., Wysota, C. N., Wang, Y., & Berg, C. J. (2021b). Predictors of negative psychosocial and health behavior impact of COVID-19 among young adults. *Health Education Research, 36*(4), 385–397. https://doi.org/10.1093/her/cyab026

Rothmann, M. J., Holton, S., Wynter, K., Rasmussen, B., & Skjøth, M. M. (2022). The impact of COVID-19 on the psychosocial well-being of nursing and midwifery staff in Denmark: A cross-sectional study. *Nordic Journal of Nursing Research.* https://doi.org/10.1177/20571585221124063

Sagherian, K., Steege, L. M., Cobb, S. J., & Cho, H. (2020). Insomnia, fatigue and psychosocial well-being during COVID-19 pandemic: A cross-sectional survey of hospital nursing staff in the United States. *Journal of Clinical Nursing.* https://doi.org/10.1111/jocn.15566

Saha, K., Torous, J., Caine, E., & De Choudhury, M. (2020). Psychosocial effects of the COVID-19 pandemic: Large-scale quasi-experimental study on social media. *Journal of Medical Internet Research, 22*(11), e22600. https://doi.org/10.2196/22600

Siow, S. L., Chuah, J. S., Roslani, A. C., Mahendran, H. A., Ratnasingam, S., & Bujang, M. A. (2022). Factors influencing the psychosocial impact of the COVID-19 pandemic on healthcare workers and their level of satisfaction towards organisational efforts. *The Medical Journal of Malaysia, 77*(2), 162–168.

Smallwood, N., Karimi, L., Bismark, M., Putland, M., Johnson, D., Dharmage, S. C., et al. (2021). High levels of psychosocial distress among Australian frontline healthcare workers during the COVID-19 pandemic: A cross-sectional survey. *General Psychiatry, 34*(5). https://doi.org/10.1136/gpsych-2021-100577

Tee, M. L., Tee, C. A., Anlacan, J. P., Aligam, K. J. G., Reyes, P. W. C., Kuruchittham, V., & Ho, R. C. (2020). Psychological impact of the COVID-19 pandemic in the Philippines. *Journal of Affective Disorders, 277*, 379–391. https://doi.org/10.1016/j.jad.2020.08.043

Theuring, S., van Loon, W., Hommes, F., Bethke, N., Mall, M. A., Kurth, T., et al. (2022). Psychosocial wellbeing of Schoolchildren during the COVID-19 Pandemic in Berlin, Germany, June 2020 to March 2021. *International Journal of Environmental Research and Public Health, 19*(16), 10103. https://doi.org/10.3390/ijerph191610103

Umeizudike, K. A., Isiekwe, I. G., Akinboboye, B. O., Aladenika, E. T., & Fadeju, A. D. (2022). Impact of the COVID-19 pandemic on the academic training and psychosocial well-being of undergraduate dental students in Nigeria. *Nigerian Journal of Clinical Practice, 25*(10), 1647. https://doi.org/10.4103/njcp.njcp_1684_21

United Nations. (2022a). *Everyone included: Social impact of COVID-19.* https://www.un.org/development/desa/dspd/everyone-included-COVID-19.html

Uribe-Restrepo, J. M., Waich-Cohen, A., Ospina-Pinillos, L., Rivera, A. M., Castro-Díaz, S., Patiño-Trejos, J. A., et al. (2022). Mental health and psychosocial impact of the COVID-19 pandemic and social distancing measures among young adults in Bogotá, Colombia. *AIMS Public Health, 9*(4), 630–643. https://doi.org/10.3934/publichealth.2022044

Von Soest, T., Kozák, M., Rodríguez-Cano, R., Fluit, S., Cortés-García, L., Ulset, V. S., et al. (2022). Adolescents' psychosocial well-being one year after the outbreak of the COVID-19 pandemic in Norway. *Nature Human Behaviour, 6*, 217–228. https://doi.org/10.1038/s41562-021-01255-w

Woodward, K. (2015). *Psychosocial studies: An introduction* (pp. 3, 4, 7, 8). New York, NY: Routledge.

Yurteri, N., & Sarigedik, E. (2021). Evaluation of the effects of the COVID-19 pandemic on sleep habits and quality of life in children. *Annals of Medical Research, 28*(1), 0186–0192. Retrieved from https://www.annalsmedres.org/index.php/aomr/article/view/331

Zainudeen, Z. T., Abd Hamid, I. J., Azizuddin, M. N. A., Bakar, F. F. A., Sany, S., Zolkepli, I. A., & Mangantig, E. (2021). Psychosocial impact of COVID-19 pandemic on Malaysian families: A cross-sectional study. *BMJ Open, 11*(8), e050523. https://doi.org/10.1136/bmjopen-2021-050523

2 "I don't know if it's Monday or October already"

A Photovoice Exploration of Psychosocial Experiences during the COVID-19 Pandemic

Sudha Shashwati, Mehar Gupta, Angela Peter, and Catherine Gomes

Introduction

COVID-19 has now established itself as one of the 21st century's significant public health crises (World Health Organization, 2020). It impacted people's physical, social, and economic well-being and caused an increase in mental health issues (Bao et al., 2020; Rajkumar, 2020). Young adults were also significantly impacted, facing social, educational, and professional disruptions (Buchanan et al., 2023). Most of these disruptions were felt most intensely during the dawn of the pandemic, when several nations instituted 'lockdowns', resulting in minimal mobility for vast populations for weeks together. The government of India instituted a 21-day lockdown on 24 March 2020, which was extended by several weeks until the end of June 2020, after which the nation started 'unlocking' though several restrictions also remained.

As remote learning and working from home became the norm even after state-instituted lockdowns were lifted, many young adults who had moved home for lockdown continued to stay with their families for safety and pragmatic reasons. While living at home might have provided relative safety from the pandemic, and some may have rejoiced in spending more time with their loved ones, home and family were not expected to provide comfort for everyone. We aimed to explore such aspects of living in lockdown and, in general, the overall lived experiences of college students in India who were compelled to return to their families due to the COVID-19 pandemic. The sudden shift back home contributed to transformations in their lives that lasted even after lockdown, which we hoped to uncover, in addition to how they navigated those transformations. In recognition of the limitations posed by conventional, text-based, or verbal qualitative research methods and the unique strengths of techniques drawn from the arts-based research (ABR) framework, we utilised the visual research method of online photovoice (OPV). ABR framework has contributed significantly to amplifying voices of the marginalised and bringing to light experiences of social inequities that might have otherwise remained invisible (e.g., Gaiha et al., 2021; Kennedy et al., 2020; Harkness & Stallworth, 2013). Our

DOI: 10.4324/9781003454984-3

study is an attempt in a similar vein. In our experience, the OPV method increased participation by expanding how participants could express or represent their experiences. Considering that we conceptualised the study during the lockdown period and conducted it during the first wave of the COVID-19 pandemic in India, we also aimed to engage in what has now been called "research resilience" (Rahman et al., 2021), elaborated in the section that follows, by making intentional methodological choices that grounded the study in the reality of the pandemic.

Methodology

Researchers all over the world encountered numerous challenges in continuing with empirical work in the aftermath of the pandemic, and qualitative research in particular, which relies on face-to-face engagement, particularly suffered in such an "unprecedented, methodologically challenging time" (Roy & Uekusa, 2020, p. 383). Researchers worldwide swiftly adapted, though, exploring several innovative and unconventional methods and new possibilities in "distance approaches to collecting qualitative data" (Taster, 2020, p. 8). The present study also involved several such intentional methodological choices in response to the pandemic context, elaborated in the sections that follow, as it was conducted during the first wave of the COVID-19 pandemic in India (July–October 2020), and the data collection coincided with the peak of the first wave.

The objective was to explore the psychosocial experiences of college students who had relocated to their families in India due to the nationwide lockdown in response to the COVID-19 pandemic. The following research questions guided the data collection:

1   What changes did returning to one's family bring in the lives of the participants?
2   How did the participants adjust to these changes?

Design

In the absence of the scope for meeting participants face-to-face, in recognition of the limitations posed by methods relying on the spoken word, and in the quest of "making the invisible visible", the visual research method of OPV was utilised. In OPV, data are gathered primarily through photographs clicked by participants, and all interactions with them, including the meaning-making of the pictures, happen in the virtual mode. These choices were made to situate the study in the pandemic context where our participants could neither meet us nor each other owing to safety guidelines and where each participant may not have had the privacy at home required to engage with conventional data collection methods like interviews. We also hoped to go beyond what an exchange of words could offer and access the ineffable, possible through images and other art forms, in this case, photographs. Furthermore, photographs have the added advantage of being young adults' currently favoured medium of telling stories about their lives, as evidenced by the rise of photograph-centric social media platforms like Instagram and Snapchat in the last decade.

Using photographs as data is not new; visual methods are popular in the ABR paradigm that began gathering steam in the 1990s, and that has been recognised as a new methodological genre (Sinner et al., 2006). It is noteworthy that the landscape of qualitative research in social sciences has fundamentally changed in the last two decades, embracing more innovative, unconventional and arts-based methods.

Our design involved the following elements: photovoice socialisation in a group setting, participants clicking photographs individually for three weeks and submitting the same, individual sense-making of a few participant-selected photographs in online interviews, and collective sense-making of all the pictures submitted in online focus group discussions.

Participants

Twenty male and female college students who had lived away from home for at least one year before the onset of the COVID-19 pandemic were invited to participate in the study through social media posts. Inclusion criteria included those who had returned home and were living at home for at least one month, had access to a camera phone and expressed no intention of moving away from home in the coming months until the study was completed. The exclusion criteria included single children, individuals living in joint families, those previously residing in a residential school, and international students. Because of the sampling method, i.e., convenience sampling, the findings cannot be generalised to the wider population. However, it is important to note that generalisation is rarely an important goal of qualitative research; instead, it is to "provide a rich, contextualised understanding of some aspect of human experience through the intensive study of particular cases" (Polit & Beck, 2010, p. 1451).

Procedure

A group orientation was conducted over video call lasting approximately 30 minutes before the data collection to establish rapport, clarify the study's purpose, take informed consent, encourage active participation, familiarise the participants with the OPV method and discuss ethical considerations involved in the same. These ethical considerations included the stipulation that participants had to secure consent from any individual appearing in their photographs. Data was then collected across three weeks, and each participant had to share 7–15 photographs with accompanying captions. Subsequently, brief online interviews were scheduled with each participant, during which they selected five photographs that best represented the stories they wished to share about their experience of moving back home for what had turned out to be an indefinite stay. These five photographs were discussed using the SHOWED framework (Wang & Redwood-Jones, 2001), addressing questions such as "What do you see here?", "What's really happening here?" and "How does this relate to our lives?" These interviews were transcribed for further analysis.

Finally, two online focus group discussions were held lasting 1.5–2 hours each that brought the participants together to view and discuss each other's photographs, thus enabling collective meaning-making of all the photographs submitted. This process is summarised in Figure 2.1. Each FGD ended with a debriefing session for the study that concluded with commemorative e-certificates presented to the participants to acknowledge their time and effort.

To ensure rigour and trustworthiness, the following steps were taken: (a) a detailed audit trail was maintained (Analysis table attached in Appendix 1) that included researchers' reflexivity and field notes, (b) analysis was done by the researchers independently to identify initial codes and then together for developing sub-themes and themes, thus engaging in a reflexive and collaborative analysis and finding inter-rater reliability of the analysis at the same time, and (c) triangulation was done by synthesising the analysis of transcripts and photographs, as illustrated in Figure 2.2.

Ethical Considerations

Without an Institutional Review Board (IRB) in the local context, we followed APA guidelines for ethical research. Informed consent was taken, and anonymity and confidentiality of the data, respecting the right to privacy and the option to withdraw at any stage were ensured throughout the study. Participants were provided with a detailed information sheet, consent forms and photo-release forms to sign, and a photovoice socialisation session was held before the beginning of data collection to have an open dialogue around issues of ethics and photography. Only codes were used throughout the study, and no identifying information was connected to any photographs or excerpts. The submitted pictures were not used for purposes other than this research, and written informed consent was obtained from those appearing in the photographs. A virtual group debriefing session was done at the end to ensure participants left the research feeling supported.

Data Analysis

The analysis stage involved the examination of photographs with accompanying narratives (captions, photo notes, and photo journals) as well as transcriptions of interviews and focus group discussions, captured in Figure 2.2. The text-based data analysis followed the six-phase approach of thematic analysis (Braun & Clarke, 2006), a flexible and accessible method for identifying and organising patterns of meaning within a dataset (Figure 2.3). Content analysis was done for the captions submitted for the photographs, which complemented the thematic analysis for the interviews and FGDs. The four researchers independently reviewed the data, identified codes, and developed themes, followed by regular online meetings to discuss differences in interpretation, promoting a collaborative and reflexive approach to qualitative data analysis. Since photographs are vulnerable to alternate readings, no research analysis was done on photographs that were submitted without captions.

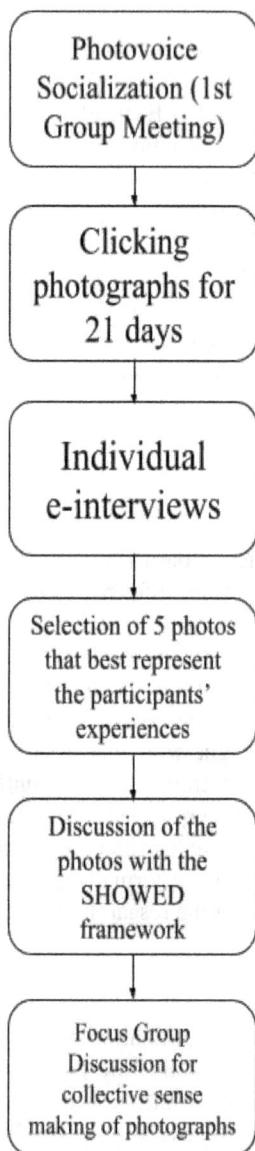

Figure 2.1 Schematic Representation of the Data Collection Process.

Findings and Discussion

The present study aimed to explore the psychosocial experiences of young adults in India during the COVID-19 pandemic after moving back home indefinitely without certainty on when restrictions on mobility would be lifted after the declaration of a nationwide lockdown. This was done using the OPV method. Since all the data

Participant Responses

Textual Data
(Transcripts)

Visual Data
(photos)

Thematic Analysis

Codes   Patterns   Sub Themes   Themes

Content Analysis

Caption and photo analysis

Triangulation of concepts based on the emerging themes from transcripts and photos

Overall Synthesis

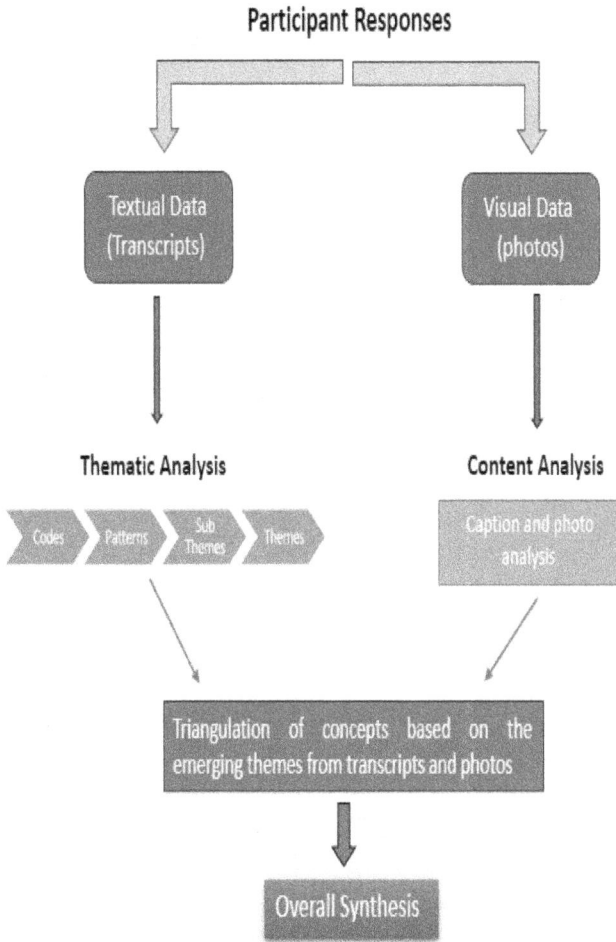

Figure 2.2 Data Analysis Stages.
Source: Adapted from Ronzi et al. (2016).

were gathered online, be it the sending of photographs or the discussion held on the photographs, both orally and via the "chat" option that allowed participants to write what they could not say out loud, participants could interact equitably and share sensitive information with us in a relatively comfortable environment. An approach such as this facilitates the exploration of subtle themes creatively, which may reveal more depth than traditional interviewing techniques. Existing literature has also deemed visual methodologies as socially situated forms of meaning-making (Gourlay, 2010), leading to a deeper and more personalised form of engagement and providing insightful triggers for discussion (Cousin, 2009). Existing literature also points to the advantage of gathering qualitative data compared to the face-to-face context, where participants have been shown to avoid eye

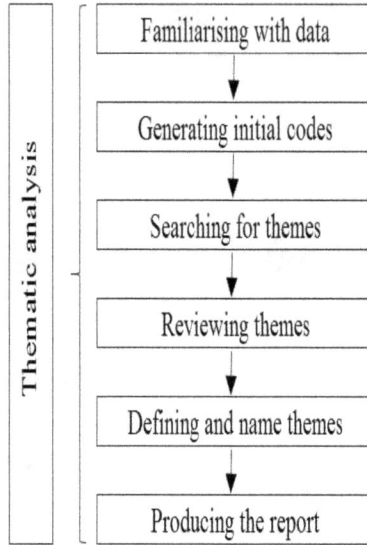

```
Thematic analysis

Familiarising with data
        ↓
Generating initial codes
        ↓
Searching for themes
        ↓
Reviewing themes
        ↓
Defining and name themes
        ↓
Producing the report
```

Figure 2.3 Thematic Analysis.

Source: Adapted from Braun and Clarke (2006) and Vaismoradi et al. (2013).

contact and speak less (Woodyatt et al., 2016; Dodds & Hess, 2020). All of these were intentional methodological choices in our study.

We generated sub-themes and themes by synthesising the text analysis (thematic analysis of interview and FGD transcripts) and photo analysis (content analysis of photo captions and photo journals) as given in Figure 2.4.

When Home Does not Feel So Homely: From Independence to Interdependence

Central to our exploration lies the notion of "home", which was demonstrated to hold different meanings for different individuals. For many participants, their college spaces and hostel rooms served as a haven, offering them an environment of independence, personal growth, and social connections. However, the sudden transition to their familial homes brought forth a clash of identities, pitting the preferred independent self against the interdependent persona demanded in the familial space. "So it becomes very chaotic, and you get scolded for anything... using the phone a lot, sitting with the laptop ...". Our findings resonate with the work of Aristovnik and colleagues, who explored the global impact of COVID-19 on college students from over 62 countries and found that increased proximity and readjustment to family dynamics led to conflicts and tensions within households (Aristovnik et al., 2020).

Through the photovoice method, we gathered glimpses of the lived experiences of the students during lockdown as they grappled with taking on caretaking

When Home Doesn't Feel So Homely: From Independence to Interdependence	*"I don't know if it's Monday or October already"*: The Pandemic Ennui	Virtual Halls, Interrupted Calls: Learning Amidst Pandemic Walls	The Pursuit of Purpose: Balancing Leisure and Productivity	No Place like Home: A Safe Haven for Uncertain Times
• The Struggles of Being with Family	• Locked in Lockdown: Going Nowhere • Tired of doing nothing, just pandemic things	• College memories: Offline over online? • E- Learning: A boon or bane?	• Free Time is a Terrible Thing to Waste • "Water, Water Everywhere, Not Any Water to Drink"	• Celebrating Family • A Little Time for Myself: Breaks as Self-Care • A Friend A Day, to Keep the Stress Away

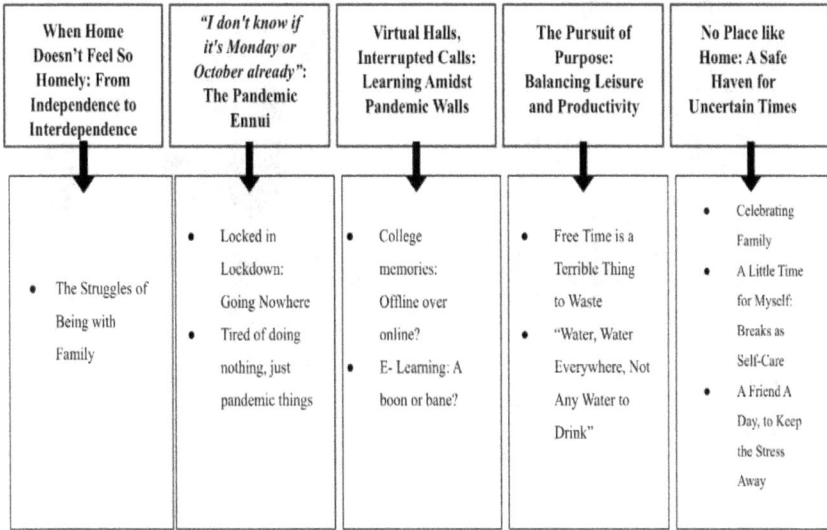

Figure 2.4 Themes and Sub-themes.

responsibilities, juggling between their virtual classes/assignments and household chores, invasion of privacy, and redefining their sense of self by engaging in hobbies/activities and spending quality time with family amidst the restraints imposed by the outside as well as the virtual world. Our participants spoke about the dominance of parental authority and how their independence was no longer theirs but controlled by others, like getting scolded for small things at home. Their photographs were pictures of the ups and downs of co-existing with the family:

> I've always hated cooking; it's like the worst thing. I hate going to the kitchen. But, being at home for so long and being forced by parents also to learn cooking and everything. I eventually landed up making a few things. So this was one of the first things I got to do in quarantine, which was something new that I would not have done otherwise.

Therefore, the experience of "home" was complex and multifaceted, and adjusting to new roles and expectations during the COVID-19 lockdown after returning home was not smooth for many of the participants (Figure 2.5).

"I don't know if it's Monday or October already": Pandemic Ennui

Participants reported feeling challenged by the sudden shift from a fast-paced world of classes, deadlines, and submissions to a slowed-down routine, lack of structure, and monotony. Due to being confined to their homes for an extended period, participants reported losing track of time and feeling bored and lethargic:

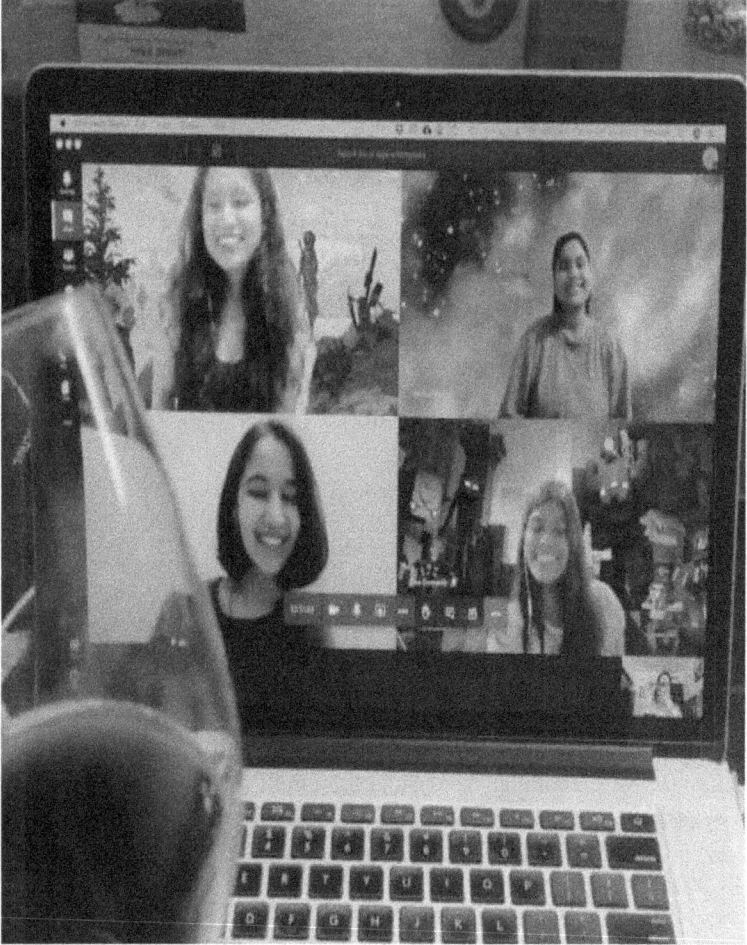

Figure 2.5 Picture by Participant.

Note. "Virtual date with my best friends".

"I don't know if it's Monday or October already, and if someone asked me the date, I'd probably say October 30th. I don't know". Another participant expressed,

> Because of all this, our brains aren't getting the same amount of stimulation that they are used to; we're having to spend our days in the same few rooms of our houses and with the same few people, so it's natural to feel more lethargic than normal as a result.

The indoor restrictions also led to feelings of isolation and confinement: "My father always tells me, I study from my bed, I eat from my bed, so he's like why are you there and I'm like I have nowhere else to go, where should I go".

According to psychotherapist Lucy Beresford, humans are "hard-wired for growth and stimulation" (Sheppard, 2021), something the pandemic, particularly the lockdown, threw into disarray. University students in different parts of the world expressed their desire to desperately want to return to their campuses because of the physical and psychological distress caused by remote learning (Birmingham et al., 2023). They reported being stressed and lacking motivation to focus on schoolwork, having sleep issues, appetite changes, and job loss

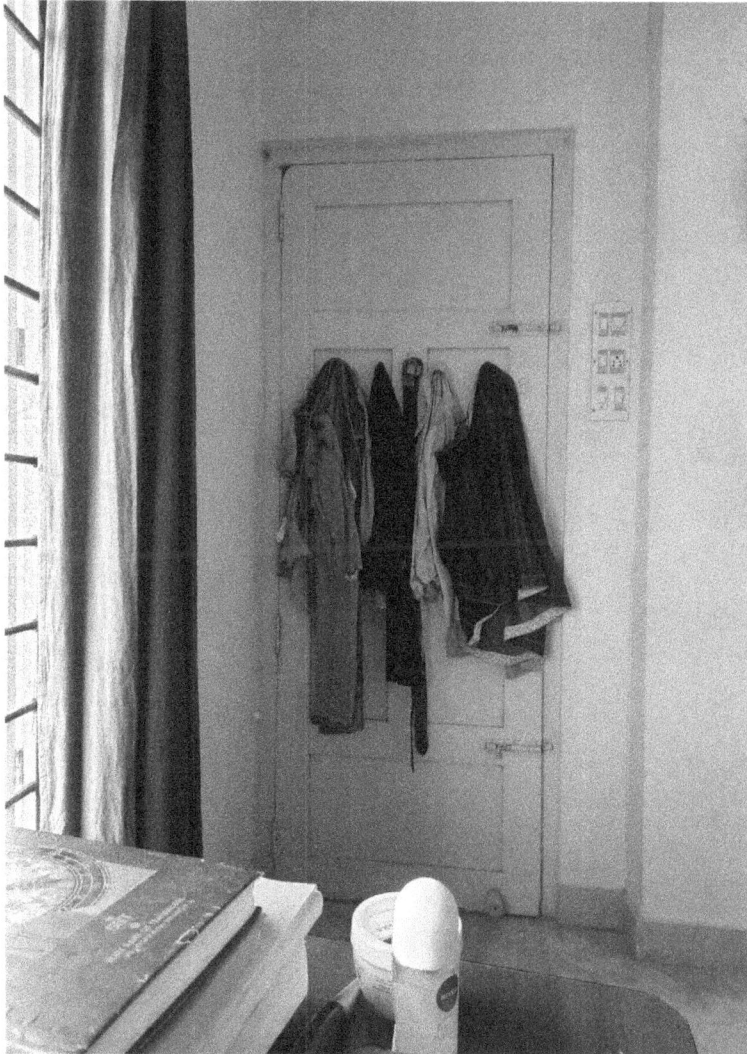

Figure 2.6 Picture by Participant.

Note. "I am sick of wearing the same clothes for half a year. I miss my clothes."

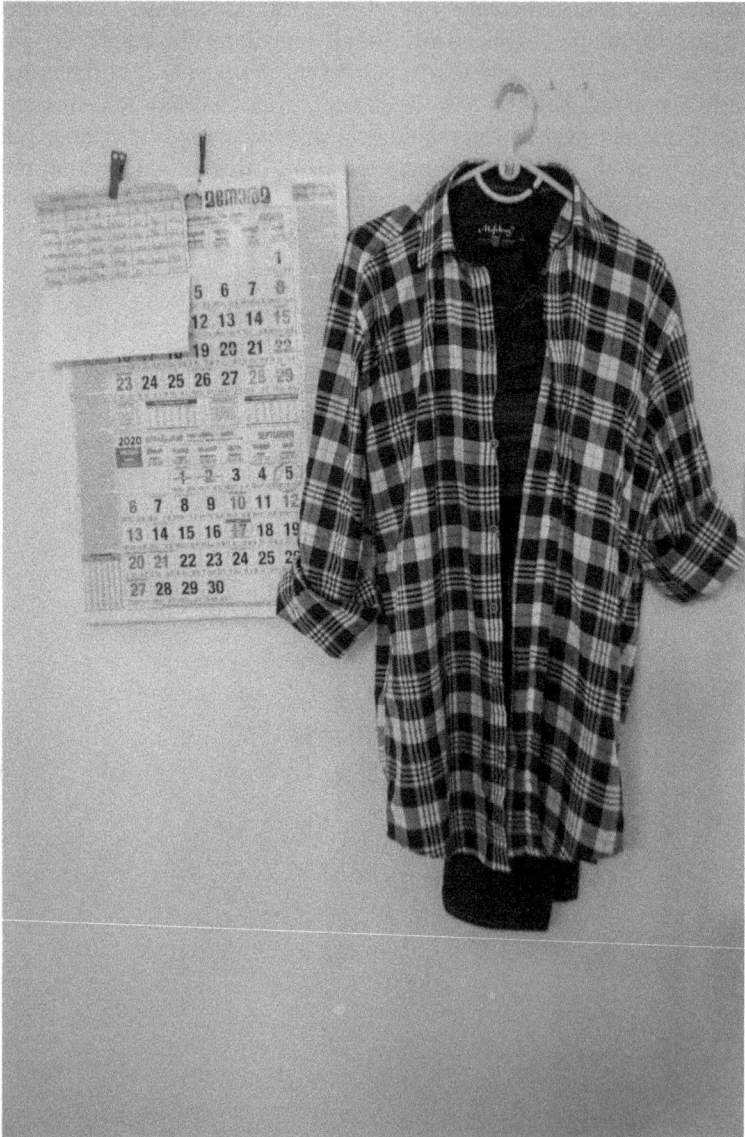

Figure 2.7 Picture by Participant.

Note. "I love to travel. Going out, meeting people, clicking some snaps, eating out. It's something that I always look forward to. On my return home, I carried clothes and a single set of casuals in case the vaccine came out. Where I'll run, I'll drive and hug tight all my friends and loved ones. Months passed, 7 to be precise; it's September. This pair doesn't seem to be going anywhere. For some more time at least."

concerns. The disruptions to academic pursuits highlighted in our study are consistent with students reporting the shift towards e-learning platforms to be extremely challenging despite flexibility and convenience (Gupta et al., 2021; Figures 2.6 and 2.7).

Virtual Halls, Interrupted Calls: Learning Amidst Pandemic Walls

Universities worldwide shifted to an online teaching mode, cancelling offline activities and events for much of 2020 (Sahu, 2020). The transition negatively impacted student lives, where many missed out on organising and participating in recreational activities/events on campus, experiencing hostel life, and attending their graduation ceremonies through a screen. Participants expressed concern about the monotony of online classes and the constant disturbances from their home environment, which further affected their ability to concentrate during lessons. One of the participants reported,

> I wake up at 8 for my 9 am classes, but till then, my home's atmosphere is not viable for taking classes. My mother would come and ask me to do the household chores like cleaning the floor or cutting the vegetables since the maid would not come. So that's going on every time.

Other studies have reported how students got bored within the first two weeks of online learning and reported considerable anxiety and mood changes due to the lack of practical exposure and the increased number of submissions and assignments (Irawan et al., 2020; Figures 2.8 and 2.9). This was reflected in some of our participants' responses as well: "… somehow teachers have the feeling that since everything is online, we don't have any work. So initially we used to get 1 assignment, but now we are getting 5, so it's best of 5". Another participant expressed concern about lack of practical knowledge and hands-on experience: "Mainly it was that it was practical based. How to use a stethoscope, how to prick a patient, how to take BP, etc. All that is not possible in online classes."

Furthermore, cancelling graduation ceremonies deprived many participants of a significant life event traditionally celebrating their hard work and accomplishments. According to Seligman's PERMA model, working towards something transcending oneself is a source of meaning, and education and career are often important sources of meaning for undergraduate students (Seligman, 2011). Studies on the extent of challenges students face during online learning have identified factors like the learning environment, distractions at home, limitations in completing certain assignments, etc. (Barrot et al., 2021). Despite the convenience of virtual learning, it is clear that the online mode of education has numerous shortcomings that need to be addressed to provide students with a fulfilling college experience.

The Pursuit of Purpose: Balancing Leisure and Productivity

Engaging with long-lost hobbies or activities that could not be pursued otherwise owing to their busy schedules before was now the main focus for many participants: "…I can do a lot of you know, drawing or painting or dancing. I don't really have time for that when I'm in Bangalore. So that is something I really loved here". Being productive allowed the participants to deal with their 'new normal'. Although there seemed to be an abundance of time during the lockdown, many

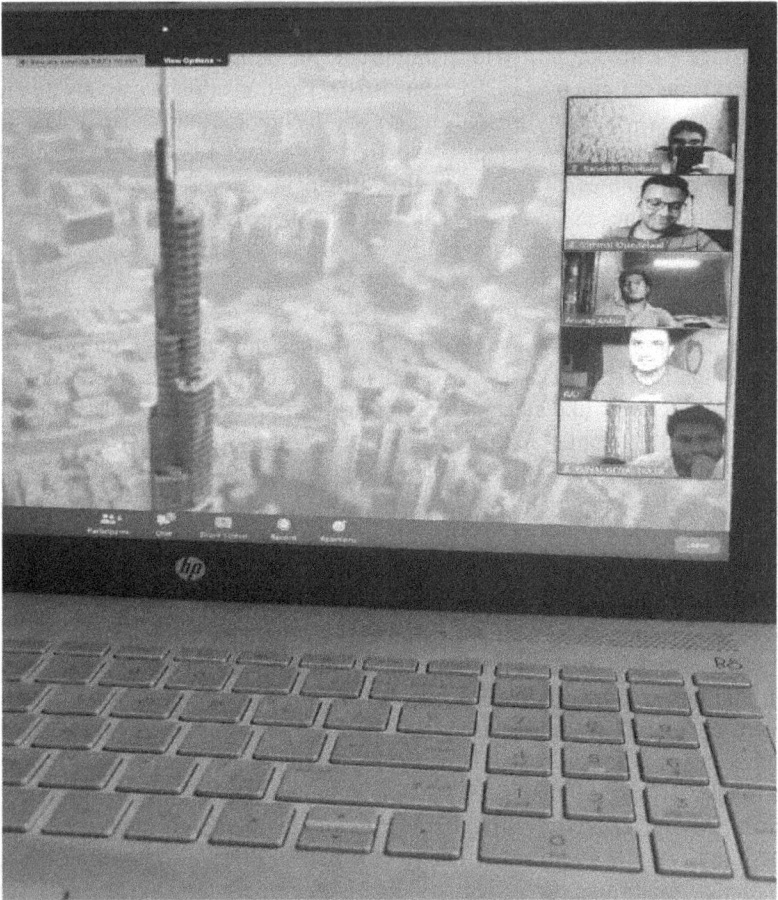

Figure 2.8 Picture by Participant.

struggled to make the most of it, which left them feeling guilty about not being more productive, something which other studies have also reported (Figures 2.10–2.13).

No Place Like Home: A Safe Haven for Uncertain Times

Home became a safe haven for many participants, and they were grateful for the company of their loved ones:

> I feel extremely grateful for all that I have, and for being safe and to be with my family in these distressing times, you know. And there are days when I really enjoy spending time with my family and they help me through my phases of doubt.

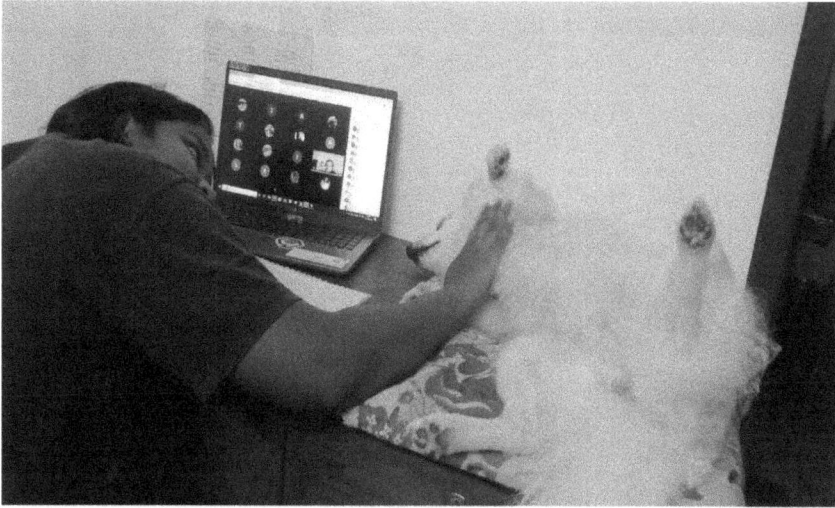

Figure 2.9 Picture by Participant.

Note. "The lockdown has made the entire life go online. Now, life is spent just in front of the 15-inch screen. Be it class, meeting or any other work."

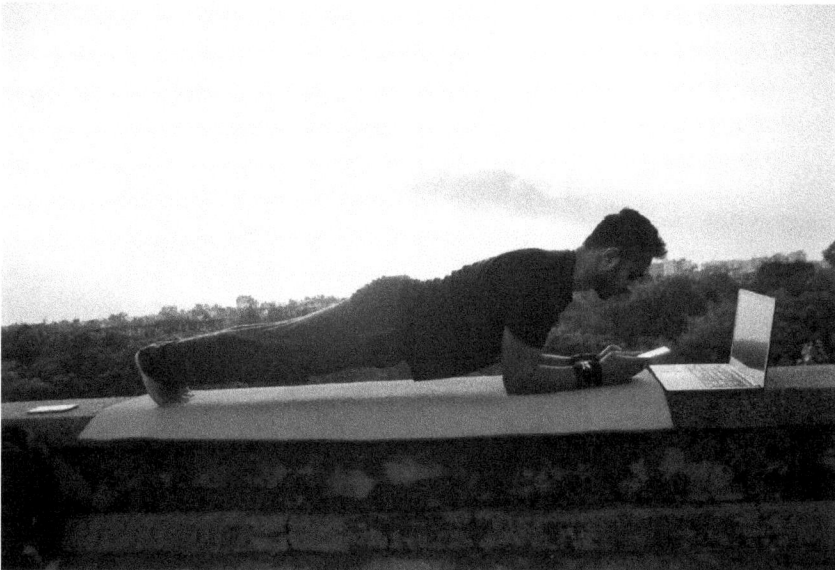

Figure 2.10 Picture by Participant.

Note. "Attending class the hard way: I started focusing on my bodily health (immunity) post-lockdown. So, this new sensation of working out while the lectures went by also happened. The boring theory lectures could be multitasked with routine workouts while the camera is off. This helped me save time and pinched me on the management basics. Pre-lockdown seemed hectic in terms of managing things. There's always a lot of time to introspect now."

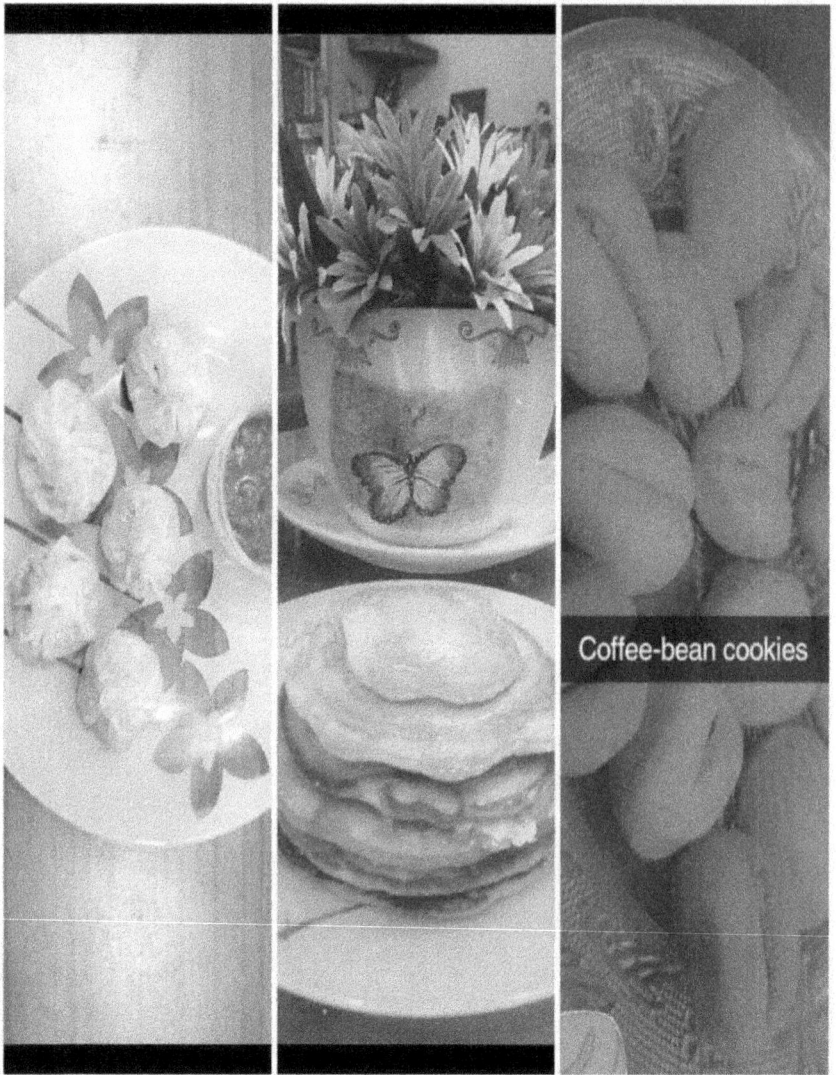

Figure 2.11 Picture by Participant.

Others expressed renewed gratitude and appreciation for their family:

> I think, I appreciate my family a little more because of this because initially all we could think of is how we are getting bored and how we don't have anything to do except for maybe scrolling our feed but like now I realise that I do have a lot of opportunities more than other people and that way I think I am more appreciative of it and I have a nice time staying with my family.

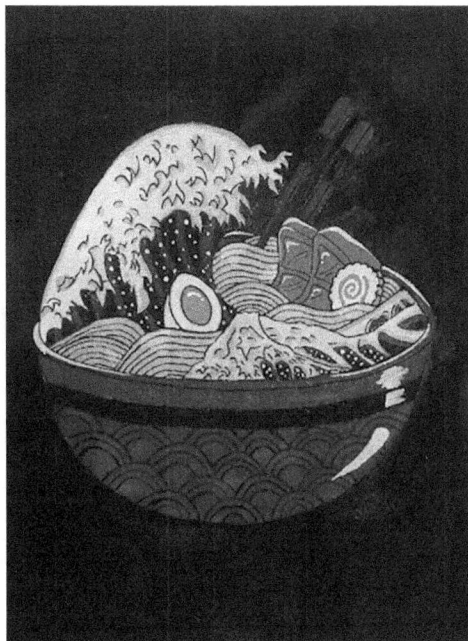

Figure 2.12 Picture by Participant.
Note. "Got back to painting."

For some participants, engaging in self-care activities and maintaining close bonds with peers through online channels helped cultivate a sense of "'safe haven" at home even more (Figure 2.14): "for me it's very important to get a little time for myself where I can do what I want to do";

> all my friends are in Delhi and i am in Dehradun so we video call everyone once a week to make sure that everyone is okay and coping up with the lockdown, with stress, classes, internships. We all have some kind of stress like siblings stress, fights, house chores, etc.

From realising that adapting to the technology-driven online mode is challenging for parents and helping them out, as illustrated in the photo note above, to making adaptations oneself in the realm of privacy and autonomy to co-exist with family members under conditions of forced confinement, this theme further highlights the diversity in participants' experiences with "home", connecting to what came up in the first theme, and brings back into focus the complex nature of what "being at home" meant for the participants.

Methodological Reflections: Notes on "Research Resilience"

Due to the dearth of qualitative studies done during the COVID-19 pandemic, specifically of a participatory nature when it comes to the Indian context, in this study,

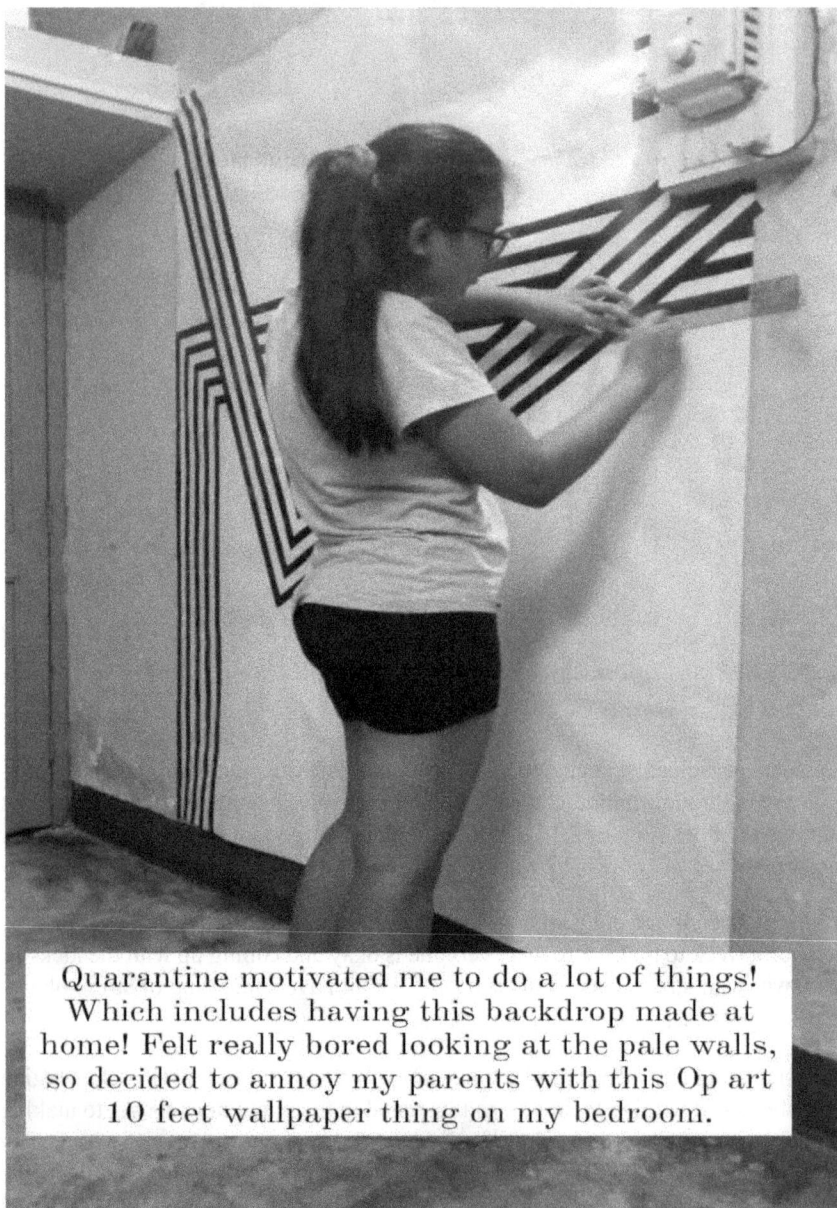

Quarantine motivated me to do a lot of things!
Which includes having this backdrop made at
home! Felt really bored looking at the pale walls,
so decided to annoy my parents with this Op art
10 feet wallpaper thing on my bedroom.

Figure 2.13 Picture by Participant.

we adopted an exploratory, qualitative design with OPV as the method of data collection, rooted in the ABR paradigm. Our methodological choices were guided by the various restrictions participants might have had to contend with, as they took part in the study from their homes and knew the significant socio-epistemic potential of pictures/photographs.

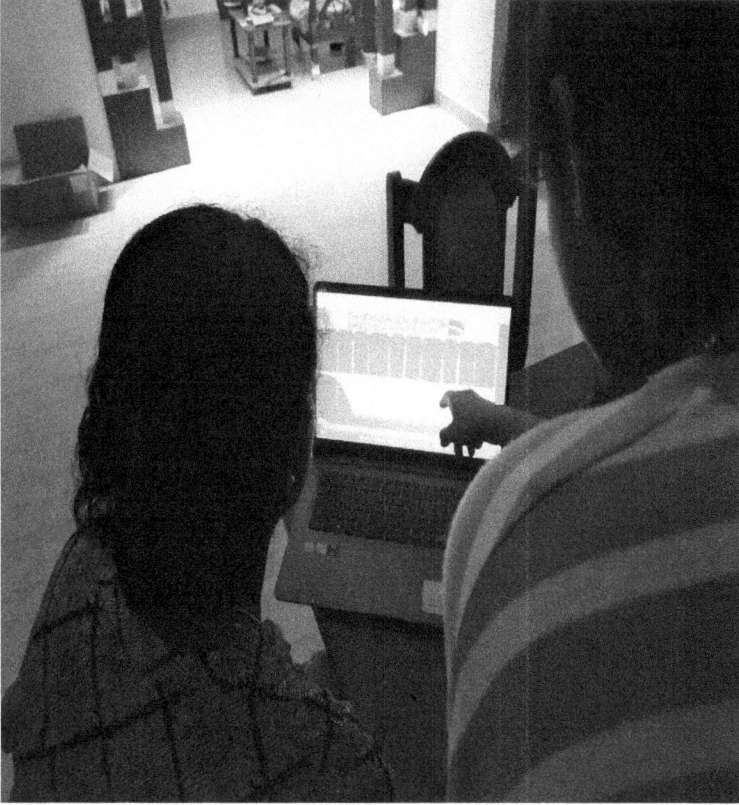

Figure 2.14 Picture by Participant.

Note. "Son, how do we join this meeting?: My parents were never into technology pre-pandemic; they are happy if there's some movie on the T.V., some tea and a handful of snacks to eat. Now that the whole system is digitised, they require our help. The frequency of calls for help and the answers to them has increased dramatically as the petty fights over it. They needed to be taught about everything, from screenshots to sending contacts via WhatsApp or joining a Zoom meeting. We did well. We're the best kids."

Based on our experience working on the present study, we argue that resilience can be integrated into the research design in qualitative research in social sciences by stretching the contours of what counts as "proper" research. The ABR paradigm, which does so, believes that the complexity of studying human behaviour demands the breaking down of the artificial separation between art and science (Butler-Kisber, 2002). We demonstrate through our work with young adults reflecting on their life and home during the pandemic using the visual research method of photovoice in the online mode the power of ABR to secure nuances of seemingly ordinary experiences that may be difficult to access via conventional representational forms or that may become catalysts of generating rich discussions with strangers (which fellow participants and researchers are, particularly in the absence of face to face interactions).

Conclusion

In the present study, we aimed to explore the psychosocial experiences of Indian college students who had been away from their families for higher studies and had to stay home for an indefinite period owing to the COVID-19 pandemic. The use of the OPV methodology allowed for in-depth exploration of the participants' lived experiences through their own eyes, as well as the potential for our participants to feel empowered throughout the research process (Wang & Burris, 1997). However, we struggled with the limitations of convenience sampling, small sample size, and short duration of data collection, because of which the empirical implications of the present study are modest. Methodologically, however, we hope this study provides examples of "research resilience" or conducting research in unprecedented crisis contexts that can be useful for future researchers. Future research in a similar context can focus on specific subgroups like international students or students from marginalised communities and could additionally compare the experiences of college students who returned home during the pandemic with those who remained in their apartments. Such research may shed light on how the pandemic affected certain student populations differently and highlight areas requiring further support.

Acknowledgement

The authors would like to express their sincere appreciation for the undergraduate students of BA Psychology (Batch of 2021) from Jesus and Mary College, Delhi University, who played a pivotal role in the data collection process for this study. This study was made possible through the collective efforts and resilience of our participants and the undergraduate students who embraced the challenges posed by the ongoing pandemic. The authors would like to acknowledge this collaborative spirit permeating every research phase.

References

Aristovnik, A., Keržič, D., Ravšelj, D., Tomaževič, N., & Umek, L. (2020). Impacts of the COVID-19 pandemic on life of higher education students: A global perspective. *Sustainability, 12*(20), 8438.

Bao, Y., Sun, Y., Meng, S., Shi, J., & Lu, L. (2020). 2019-nCoV pandemic: Address mental health care to empower society. *Lancet (London, England), 395*(10224), e37–e38.

Barrot, J., Llenares, I. I., & Del Rosario, L. S. (2021). Students' online learning challenges during the pandemic and how they cope with them: The case of the Philippines. *Education and Information Technologies, 26*(6), 7321–7338.

Birmingham, W. C., Wadsworth, L. L., Lassetter, J. H., Graff, T. C., Lauren, E., & Hung, M. (2023). COVID-19 lockdown: Impact on college students' lives. *Journal of American College Health, 71,* 879–893.

Braun, V., & Clarke, V. (2006). Using thematic analysis in psychology. *Qualitative Research in Psychology, 3*(2), 77–101.

Buchanan, D., Hargreaves, E., & Quick, L. (2023). Schools closed during the pandemic: Revelations about the well-being of 'lower-attaining' primary-school children. *Education, 51,* 1077–1090.

Butler-Kisber, L. (2002). Artful portrayals in qualitative inquiry: The road to found poetry and beyond. *Alberta Journal of Educational Research, 48*(3). https://doi.org/10.11575/ajer.v48i3.54930

Cousin, G. (2009). *Researching learning in higher education: An introduction to contemporary methods and approaches.* Routledge, UK.

Dodds, S., & Hess, A. C. (2020). Adapting research methodology during COVID-19: Lessons for transformative service research. *Journal of Service Management, 32*(2), 203–217.

Gaiha, S. M., Salisbury, T. T., Usmani, S., Koschorke, M., Raman, U., & Petticrew, M. (2021). Effectiveness of arts interventions to reduce mental-health-related stigma among youth: A systematic review and meta-analysis. *BMC Psychiatry, 21*, 364.

Gourlay, L. (2010). Multimodality, visual methodologies and higher education. In *New approaches to qualitative research* (pp. 96–104). Routledge, UK.

Gupta, S., Dabas, A., Swarnim, S., & Mishra, D. (2021). Medical education during COVID-19 associated lockdown: Faculty and students' perspective. *Medical Journal, Armed Forces India, 77*(Suppl 1), S79–S84.

Harkness, S. S., & Stallworth, J. (2013). Photovoice: Understanding high school females' conceptions of mathematics and learning mathematics. *Educational Studies in Mathematics, 84*, 329–347.

Irawan, A., Dwisona, D., & Lestari, M. (2020). Psychological impacts of students on online learning during the COVID-19 pandemic. *KONSELI: Jurnal Bimbingan dan Konseling (E-Journal), 7*, 53–60. https://doi.org/10.24042/kons.v7i1.6389.

Kennedy, H., Marley, M., Torres, K., Edelblute, A., & Novins, D. (2020). "Be creative, and you will reach more people": Youth's experiences participating in an arts-based social action group aimed at mental health stigma reduction. *Arts & Health, 12*(1), 23–37.

Polit, D. F., & Beck, C. T. (2010). Generalisation in quantitative and qualitative research: Myths and strategies. *International Journal of Nursing Studies, 47*(11), 1451–1458.

Rahman, S. A., Tuckerman, L., Vorley, T., & Gherhes, C. (2021). Resilient research in the field: Insights and lessons from adapting qualitative research projects during the COVID-19 pandemic. *International Journal of Qualitative Methods, 20*, 160940692110161.

Rajkumar, R. P. (2020). COVID-19 and mental health: A review of the existing literature. *Asian Journal of Psychiatry, 52*, 102066.

Ronzi, S., Pope, D., Orton, L., & Bruce, N. (2016). Using photovoice methods to explore older people's perceptions of respect and social inclusion in cities: Opportunities, challenges and solutions. *SSM-Population Health, 2*, 732–745.

Roy, R., & Uekusa, S. (2020). Collaborative autoethnography: "Self-reflection" as a timely alternative research approach during the global pandemic. *Qualitative Research Journal, 20*(4), 383–392.

Sahu, P. (2020). Closure of universities due to coronavirus disease 2019 (COVID-19): Impact on education and mental health of students and academic staff. *Cureus, 12*(4), e7541.

Seligman, M. (2011). *Flourish: A visionary new understanding of happiness and well-being.* Washington, DC: PsycNET.

Sheppard, T. (2021, December 14). *COVID-19 | Why doing nothing makes you feel tired | Data driven investor.* Medium.

Sinner, A., Leggo, C., Irwin, R. L., Gouzouasis, P., & Grauer, K. (2006). Arts-based educational research dissertations: Reviewing the practices of new scholars. *Canadian Journal of Education, 29*(4), 1223–1270.

Taster, M. (2020). Editorial: Social science in a time of social distancing. *LSE Impact Blog, 23*.

Vaismoradi, M., Turunen, H., & Bondas, T. (2013). Qualitative descriptive study. *Nursing & Health Sciences, 15,* 398–405.

Wang, C., & Burris, M. A. (1997). Photovoice: Concept, methodology, and use for participatory needs assessment. *Health Education & Behaviour, 24*(3), 369–387.

Wang, C. C., & Redwood-Jones, Y. A. (2001). Photovoice ethics: Perspectives from Flint photovoice. *Health Education & Behaviour, 28*(5), 560–572.

Woodyatt, C., Finneran, C., & Stephenson, R. (2016). In-person versus online focus group discussions. *Qualitative Health Research, 26*(6), 741–749.

World Health Organization. (2020, February 12). *Covid-19 public health emergency of international concern (PHEIC) global research and innovation forum.* World Health Organization.

Appendix 1

Analysis Table

Codes, Themes and Sub-themes

Themes	Sub-themes	Codes
When Home Doesn't Feel so Homely: From Independence to Interdependence	**The Struggles of Being with Family**	• Lack of Freedom at home • Lack of Privacy at home • Increased interference at home • Monotony and frustration of living with the same people lead to fighting • Lack of time for self at home • Having to be answerable for every action • Usually feel like a guest in my own house post-return • Learning to cook during quarantine due to parental pressure despite hating it • Getting scolded for small things at home
***"I don't know if it's Monday or October already"*: The Pandemic Ennui**	**Locked in Lockdown: Going Nowhere**	• Restrictions imposed due to the lockdown • All activities confined to the bed • No scope for planning a vacation • Missing street food • Missing out on birthday celebrations • Miss partying, social interaction
	Tired of Doing Nothing, Just Pandemic Things	• Losing track of time due to lockdown • Monotony due to virtual mode and same routine • Lack of fixed routine at home • Excited at first but now family time is monotonous
Virtual Halls, Interrupted Calls: Learning Amidst Pandemic Walls	**College Memories: Offline Over Online?**	• Missing out on college events due to transition to virtual mode • Loss of anticipated, positive experiences at college • Disappointments due to missing out on college life • Missing hostel charm and warmth

(Continued)

(Continued)

Themes	Sub-themes	Codes
	E-Learning: A Boon or Bane?	• Disruption/interference during online classes • Negative impact of online classes on daily routine • Realisation that working online was a tough task • Dislike for online classes • Multi-tasking with online classes and helping with chores • Online classes impacting education negatively • Increased workload causing stress • Restricted movement at home • Irritation and difficulty in adapting to online shift • Increased workload due to college moving online • Online classes impacting education: lack of practical knowledge
The Pursuit of Purpose: Balancing Leisure and Productivity	Free Time Is a Terrible Thing to Waste	• Learning new skills during quarantine • Lockdown as a time for hobbies • Trying new courses • Being trapped in the vicious cycle of productivity • Engaging in hobbies to "kill time" • Inculcating skills to distract oneself from excessive screen time • Lockdown- an opportunity to indulge in abandoned hobbies
	"Water, Water Everywhere, Not Any Water to Drink"	• Lack of time for self at home • Inconvenience due to lack of space at home • A sense of loss of freedom • A sense of invasion of privacy • Having to be answerable for every action.
No Place like Home: A Safe Haven for Uncertain Times	Celebrating Family	• It is important to look at the brighter side of things. • Gratitude to be with family and acknowledgement of privilege. • Family time to improve bonding. • Enjoying time with cousins. • Family is the source of happiness. • Gratitude for being able to celebrate festivals at home • Good food available at home, unlike college • Realisation that online is tough for parents • Realisation that one should celebrate life • Happiness in meeting siblings after a long time • Important to look at the bright side of things • Grateful for being safe at home with parents

(*Continued*)

(Continued)

Themes	Sub-themes	Codes
	A Little Time for Myself: Breaks as Self-Care	• Taking necessary breaks to bust stress and boost energy • Taking out time for self when overwhelmed with work • Discovering new things about oneself • Realisation that enjoyment lies in the little things • Acknowledgement of one's own freedom • Gratitude and acknowledgement of privilege
	A Friend a Day, to Keep the Stress Away	• Video call with friends as a way to deal with overburdening stress • Talking to friends lightens mood • Talking to friends helps in gaining perspective about one's issues • Talking to friends helps in finding solutions to problems

3 Impact and Challenges of COVID-19

A Situational Analysis

Abhishek Mishra, Shachi Mishra, Jayant Kumar, and Anil Kumar

Introduction

This research comes under the domain of "Sociology of Pandemic", the term coined by the British Sociologist Philip Strong (1990) in his paper on "epidemic psychology". He tried to explain the epidemics of fear and moralisation of social stigma among AIDS patients (Ward, 2020; Prasad, Kumar, and Srivastava, 2021). It is a fact and well-grounded reality that the pandemic is a medical anomaly and a significant societal risk. The various social philosophers have analysed risks and fears posed by pandemics to the people "Risk Society" (Beck, 1992), "digital risk society" (Lupton, 2016), Conspiracy Theories (Popper, 1966, 1972; Machiavelli, 1532; Coady, 2003, 2021), "unwarranted conspiracy theories" (Keeley, 1999), "Testimonial Injustice" (Fricker, 2007). COVID-19 has explored a new challenge as a failure of the interventions in the field of public health designed by the technocrats based on conceptions to make personal benefits far from reality (Freire, 1970; Papa et al., 2006). It has been observed that with the nationwide social lockdown and the shutting down of almost livelihood-generating activities, the citizens faced a drastic change in their daily lives. The country's economic progress started pulling down (Stephanie & Dylan, 2020; Ambika et al., 2021, p. 2).

On the other hand, during the lockdown, environmental improvement was obvious due to the decline in daily activities, which reduced all kinds of pollution, halting the degradation of nature (Ambika et al., 2021).

Contemporary society is going through the condition of "Risk Society". The term was used by Ulrich Beck (1992) and Anthony Giddens (1999). Beck observed the process of modernisation, which dissolved the feudal social structure in the nineteenth century and shaped the upgraded social system, i.e., industrial society. However, the modernisation process in the contemporary world is dissolving industrial society and another form of modernity is coming into being (Beck, 1992) called a second modernity or reflective modernity. He mentioned that risk distribution history is reflected in the class pattern, where wealth is accumulated at the topmost in the class hierarchy and the risks at the bottom part of the population (Beck, 1992). Beck argues that many health risks are the outcome of human action in the modernising processes that created risks for individuals and society; for example, all kinds of pollution, chemically contaminated

DOI: 10.4324/9781003454984-4

food, and epidemics of bacterial infections caused by the inappropriate consumption of antibiotics are the results of over exercise of modern techniques even forced by the experts for profit making. On this ground, we could understand the COVID-19 period as a transition from civil society to a new era distinguished by technological hazards, distributing "bads" (pollution, contamination, and other by-products of production) considered preventable. Giddens (1991) emphasises the political aspects of risk and considers it (modernity) as a risk culture for society due to people losing their trust in experts.

Lupton (2016) observed the experience of the new form of digital technologies in social life and social institutions affecting both public and personal life due to increasing monitoring by digital surveillance devices and sensors, creating a field of risk inquiry that might be termed as a "digital risk society". In the contemporary world, such forms of digital technology are used by conspirators to create fake information to create fear and uncertainty in society.

Conspiracy theories refer to a theory or explanation that features a conspiracy among a group of agents as a central ingredient. The term "conspiracy theory" was first made famous in the 1950s by Sir Karl Popper (an Austrian-British philosopher). Until then, conspiracy theories have had a bad reputation among social scientists. Conspiracy theories are, in general, not only producing wrong information, which are the products of irrationality. The narration of such theories is also unsafe for the individuals or the targeted population; hence, such activities or thoughts could be treated as a problem, which might be resolved, or at least moderated by the social scientists in general or the psychologists, public health experts and even philosophers from any branch of knowledge, through interventions.

The unique pandemic condition known as COVID-19 was brought on by a recently discovered virus called Severe Acute Respiratory Syndrome Coronavirus 2. SARS-CoV-2 began as an epidemic in mainland China, with the World Health Organization (WHO) receiving its first report on 31 December 2019, from Wuhan in the Hubei region (Andrews et al., 2020). The WHO classified the coronavirus outbreak of 2019 and declared it a pandemic on 11 March 2020 (WHO, 2022a). Although the early cases of SARS-CoV-2 have been linked to the Wuhan South China Seafood Market, the origin and source of the virus are still unknown. Since bat SARS-CoV-like coronaviruses 2 and SARS-CoV-2 are similar, it is most likely that bats act as reservoir hosts for the species that gave rise to them (Andersen et al., 2020). As of 11 October 2022, India ranked third globally in terms of COVID-19-related mortality (528,822) and second globally in terms of reported confirmed cases (44,616,394) after the United States and Brazil (Worldometer, 2022). Conspiracy theories were frequently discussed as a threat to public safety and even as a threat to democracy itself during the COVID-19 era (Pauly, 2020). It is an injustice to those whose opinions were typified by conspiracy theories; another negative effect was noted. Miranda Fricker (2007) dubbed this phenomenon "testimonial injustice" (Coady, 2021). Brian Keeley (1999) defined it as "unwarranted conspiracy theories" that evolved from Popper's work as conspiracies in the literature on philosophy. Popper posed the difficulty of demarcating between science and pseudoscience in the context of conspiracy theories, whereas Keeley addressed the issue of distinguishing between warranted and unwarranted conspiracy theories (Pauly, 2020).

The first case of COVID-19 was reported on 27 January 2020 from Kerala, a southern Indian State, by a 20-year-old female medical student. She returned from Wuhan, the city of China, the pandemic's epicentre (Andrews et al., 2020). The COVID-19 pandemic spread to Uttar Pradesh (UP) in March 2020. The first case of COVID-19 in UP was reported on 5 March 2020 from the Ghaziabad district by someone who had travelled to Iran (Andrews et al., 2020). The second case of COVID-19 was reported from Agra (popularly known as Taj Nagari) in UP. The first cases of COVID-19 in the Ballia district were reported on 10 May 2020. Those who had travel history to Ahmedabad tested positive. The government of UP has developed a unified state COVID-19 web portal (http://upcovid19tracks.in) designed to capture all information related to surveillance, testing, treatment, contact tracing, home isolation, and admission in health care facilities, containment zones and details of other field activities for COVID-19 patients. Regular skill enhancement training for the health staff was provided to ensure data quality and its management at the district level. Data availability in a digital form facilitated decentralised and granular analysis for quick decision-making and response. The portal also had interoperability with the Government of India portal. The Government of UP has made it mandatory for all the district government and private healthcare facilities to upload all COVID-19-related data on this portal. Under the supervision of District Surveillance Officers (DSO Panel, 2022) and Chief Medical Officer (CMO), a dedicated data entry operator was assigned to every administrative block of the district to feed data regularly. Data feeding on the "upcovid19track" portal was done and analysed daily by the Integrated Disease Surveillance Programme (IDSP) Unit established at the district level.

It was observed during the literature review that a comparative situational analysis of the first, second and third waves of the COVID-19 pandemic was done at the level of countries and states like South Korea (Seong et al., 2021), India (Sarkar et al., 2021), Australia (Begum et al., 2022), Europe, United States (James et al., 2021) but it has not been done for the underdeveloped cities and farfetched districts from the state capital regions in the developing countries like India. Hence, we conducted this study intending to analyse the situation of COVID-19 from February 2020 to February 2022 and to assess the evolution of COVID-19 preparedness in the Ballia district of UP, India a "C Grade City" of the state (Govt. of UP, 2022) with mid-year population of 3,655,474 for the year 2022 (Ballia Population, 2021/2022), a comparatively underdeveloped district of UP.

Methodology

Based on the overall development, the government of UP has categorised all its administrative districts into A, B, and C Categories (Govt. of UP, 2022). Ballia, a "C Category" district, is comparatively less developed than UP, India's category A and B cities. Hence, we selected the Ballia district for our cross-sectional study. Our study period is from the beginning of preparation for the pandemic in Ballia to the end of the third wave, i.e., February 2020 to 2022. We conducted key informant interviews and reviewed surveillance reports, upcovid19track portal data, CoWin portal (a dedicated portal for feeding of COVID-19 vaccination data developed by the government of India), reports from private health facilities, and patient treatment cards, records from the district health department office. Key informants were interviewed using a semi-structured questionnaire. Data related to COVID-19 cases and vaccination were downloaded in an Excel file, arranged, and extracted using a data extraction plan. Attendants of deceased patients were interviewed telephonically using a data collection tool for information related to the place of death and hospital admission. Data related to deceased cases not registered on the upcovid19track portal is obtained using a data extraction table from the records of the district Disaster Management Cell office. All the data was tabulated, entered into Microsoft Excel, and analysed using Epi-Info 7.2.5 (CDC, 2022). We analysed data by time (epidemic curve), place (area-specific positivity rate), and person (attack rate, testing modality, and CFR by age). Proportions were calculated for case type and facilities reporting COVID-19 cases. We maintained the confidentiality of the data and did not collect any personal identifiers. All the administrative approval for the study and publication is obtained from competent district-level health authorities.

Result

COVID-19: 1st Wave Situational Analysis and Preparedness

The first case of COVID-19 was reported in Ballia on 10 May 2020. From 20 June 2020, the cases of COVID-19 have increased exponentially in the district, and after 262 days, the cases of COVID-19 started declining from 27 January 2021 onwards. During the first wave of COVID-19 in Ballia from 10 May 2020 to 27 January 2021, 8,007 cases were reported with an AR of 0.002 and a sample positivity rate (SPR) of 3.2 per 100 samples. Of the total COVID cases in the first wave, 69% were male. Among the total cases reported, 7% belong to the paediatric age group of 0–15 years. Most cases were from the rural areas of Ballia district, 85%. Out of 8,007 COVID-19-positive cases reported, about 42% of the cases were picked up on random sampling, 27% cases were asymptomatic contacts of COVID-positive cases, 12% were Symptomatic cases, 17% cases were detected in various field activities, 1% cases were detected among the patients planning for various medical procedures like surgeries, dialysis, radiotherapy, and daycare procedures. Among national and international travellers of Ballia, 0.6% tested positive for COVID-19.

During first wave of the COVID-19, the most affected area of Ballia district was Hanumanganj block with SPR of 7.85 per 100 followed by Ballia City (PR= 5.58), Gadwar (PR=3.13), Beruwarbari (PR=3.11), Siar (PR=3), Rasara (PR=2.8), Pandah (PR=2.8), Belahari (PR=2.7), Chilkahar (PR=2.7), Revati (PR=2.7), Nawanagar (PR=2.6), Bansdeeh (PR=2.6), Nagara (PR=2.5), Maniyar (PR=2.4), Murli

Chapara (PR=2.2), Dubahad (PR=1.9), Sohaon (PR=1.9) and Bairiya (PR=1.7). Among total COVID-19-positive cases during the first wave in Ballia, 41% tested positive by Rapid Antigen Test, 55% tested positive by Real-Time Polymerase Chain Reaction (RT-PCR) test, and 4% tested positive by Cartridge Based Nucleic Acid Amplification Test (CB-NAAT) and TrueNat (chip-based, point of care, rapid molecular test). All COVID-19 cases during the first wave in Ballia were reported from 77 Health Care Institutions, of which 44% were Government Institutions and 56% were private facilities. Of the COVID-19 cases, 95% were reported from government institutions, and 5% were from private institutions. Among Government Institutions, the maximum number of COVID-19 cases (49%) were reported by the "Institute of Medical Sciences-Banaras Hindu University" (IMS-BHU), followed by "Ballia Antigen Lab and District Hospital Ballia" (41%). Most of the cases from Private Institutions were reported from Heritage (0.9%) and Apex (0.5%) hospitals of Varanasi city. The average time taken to get the RT PCR result for an individual of Ballia was 1.5 Days during the first wave of COVID-19. There was a total of 127 deaths reported during 1st COVID-19 wave, out of which 107 were registered on the "upcovid19track Portal" and 20 deceased cases were reported to the administration after the announcement of compensation for COVID-19 death cases by the government, with case fatality rate (CFR) of 13 per 1,000 positive cases, the first death was reported on 28 June 20, out of total deceased 95 were male and 28 were female. Among reported deceased cases, three were children in the age group of 5–13 years. Among the deceased, 53% are senior citizens aged 60 years and above, with an age-specific CFR of 6.7 per 100 positive cases and a SPR of 4.4. All the deceased cases during the first COVID-19 wave expired at health facilities. Of the total reported cases in the first COVID-19, 74% were home-isolated, and 26% were admitted to Health Facilities (Table 3.1).

Given the increasing number of cases during the first wave of COVID-19, certain preventive interventions were taken up by the health authorities of Ballia with the support of the District Administration. The first RT-PCR sampling for the COVID-19 test was done on 6 February 2020 and sent to King George Medical University, Lucknow, followed by the initiation of a Rapid Antigen Test in the district on 14 July 2020. As the pandemic enters India, the Central Government has steadfastly led the response and management strategy for COVID-19, focusing on managing the pandemic in the States and Districts. In close coordination and integral collaboration, the State governments have implemented the centre-led policies and interventions. Many have also designed customised, innovative measures to fight the pandemic. Others emulate these, facilitating the wider implementation of regional ideas and best practices. The Government of UP has taken various initiatives in this direction. To strengthen the case management and surveillance, the surveillance committees called Nigrani and Mohalla Samities, along with a 24×7 Integrated Covid Command Centre, were established in the district on 01 May 20 and 18 July 2020 respectively, as per the instructions from the state with representation of all relevant departments to address the rising number of positive cases. The Nigrani Samitis were established in rural areas, and Mohalla Samitis were established in urban areas, including cities and census towns of the district, to identify, isolate and test any travellers coming into their village or Mohalla from the endemic areas of the country (MoHFW, 2022). The Integrated Covid Control and Command Centre (ICCC), headed by Chief Development Officer Ballia, ensures effective coordination among relevant departments for Non-Pharmaceutical Interventions. It also facilitates prompt referral of COVID-19 patients to the appropriate level of dedicated COVID-19 facilities. The ICCC's main task is coordinating with all the stakeholders to ensure prompt testing of symptomatic patients and contacts, intimation of laboratory status, facilitation of transport and facility allocation in case of admission, and regular follow-up of cases under home isolation. The ICCC functions through various cells:

1 **Home Isolation Cell:** Health information of COVID-19-positive patients was obtained by the Home Isolation cell telephonically after the physician assigned a COVID-19-positive patient home isolation. This cell works through 132 people in two shifts. In this cell, the people of the education and health department have been engaged in calling and consulting doctors. The home isolation cell is used to take information daily for SPO2 level, symptoms, information about receipt of medicine kit, information about the visit of rapid response team (RRT) from the health department, and information about the installation of the Arogya Setu App. If the patients needed it, this cell helped them get admitted to the hospital. This cell is functioning through 02 helpline numbers in Ballia.

2 **Hospital and Public Grievance Redressal Cell**: This cell receives general public grievances related to COVID-19 through 04 helpline numbers, transfers them to the concerned departments, and receives feedback on those complaints. This cell solved the problem of patients by taking information and feedback about the status of the patients admitted to the dedicated COVID-19 hospitals. This cell worked in 03 shifts through one nodal officer and a team of 12 people.

3 **Patient Shifting Cell**: The main function of this cell was to get the COVID-19-positive patients admitted to COVID-19-specific hospitals by ambulance by coordinating with the hospital and public grievance cell and home isolation cell. Two doctors were operating on this cell. This cell also operated a WhatsApp group for quick information and action.

4 **Vaccination Cell**: This cell was established to motivate the persons who had taken the first dose of the COVID-19 vaccine to get the second one and to coordinate with various government departments involved in mobilising people for vaccination. This cell was functioning through 09 nodal officers and 80 callers.

5 **COVID Counselling Cell**: With doctors' help, this cell provided advisory facilities related to COVID-19. Additionally, this cell also provided psychological counselling to the patient as well as their family members.

6 **Nigrani Samiti Cell**: This cell reviewed the work of monitoring committees (Nigrani Samities); it obtained information on any new traveller who arrived in the allocated area, their sampling, isolation, RRT visit, and availability of medicine kit.

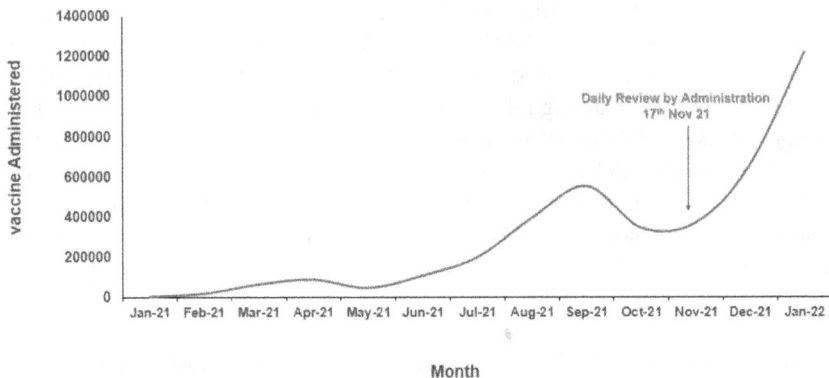

Figure 3.1 Impact of Daily Review Meeting on Vaccination.

Three dedicated healthcare care units were established for isolation and better management of COVID-19-affected individuals, out of which one was named L1 facilities were facilities for isolation and management of mild COVID-19 cases were made available, and two healthcare units named L2 facilities (Basantpur & Phephana). The facilities for invasive and non-invasive ventilation were made available. Moderate to severe cases were admitted in these facilities. A 12-bed ward and an operation theatre (OT) were also reserved at the district women's hospital for the management of COVID-19-affected pregnant women. Given the increasing number of cases in the district, the RT-PCR lab was established on 3 October 2020. Overall, during the first wave of the COVID-19 epidemic, a continuous epidemic curve was observed (Figure 3.1). For effective control of the SARS-CoV-2 virus, sanitisation activities were also initiated in the district by the Panchayati Raj Institution (PRI). The health department shared a line list of daily positive cases with Nagarpalika and PRI, following which the sanitisation activities with 1% Sodium hypochlorite (Directorate of Medical & Health Services, UP, 2022, October 14) solution were done in the residence and vicinity of COVID-19 cases.

Near the end of the first COVID-19 wave, the mass COVID-19 vaccination campaign was started in the district. Along with the other districts of India and UP, the COVID-19 Vaccination was started for healthcare workers on 16 January 2021. The next phase of the vaccination drive begins on 1 March 2021 for all the residents of Ballia over the age of 60 and residents between the ages of 45 and 60 who have one or more qualifying comorbidities; by the beginning of May 2021, the COVID vaccination was started for all the residents of Ballia aged 18 years and above (Koshy, 2021). From 27 January 2021 onward, the number of COVID-19 cases reported in Ballia was in binary numbers, indicating the end of the first wave. However, the number of cases again started rising from 21 March 2021 onwards, which was the beginning of the second wave of COVID-19 in the district (Figure 3.2).

1st Wave

2nd Wave

3rd Wave

>5 %

4.9 to 4 %

3.9 to 3 %

2.9 to 2 %

< 2 %

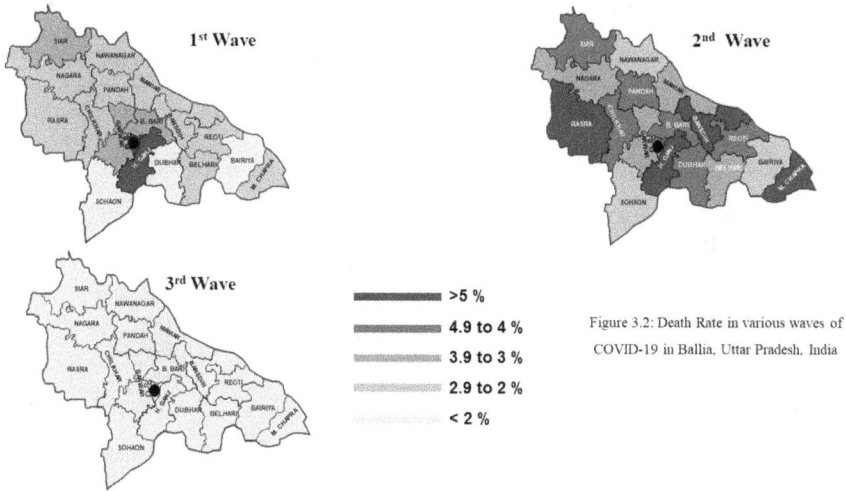

Figure 3.2: Death Rate in various waves of
COVID-19 in Ballia, Uttar Pradesh, India

Figure 3.2 Death Rate in Various Waves of COVID-19.

COVID-19: Second Wave Situational Analysis and Preparedness

The second wave of the Novel coronavirus epidemic was declared on 22 March 2021 in the district, during which 13,461 COVID-19-positive cases were reported in just three months (from 20 March 2021 to 19 June 2021) during this period an average of 137 cases were reported per day in the district with AR of 0.004 and SPR of 4.3. During the second wave of COVID-19, about 93% of cases were reported from rural areas and 7% from urban areas of Ballia district. Out of the total cases in the second wave, 68% were male and 32% female. Among the total cases reported, 6.5% belong to the paediatric age group, i.e., 0–15 years. Out of a total of 13,461 positive cases reported, most of the cases 16% were picked up on random sampling, 18% cases were asymptomatic contacts of COVID-19 positive cases, 18% were Symptomatic cases during various public health field activities, 47% cases were detected, 0.7% cases were detected among the patients planning for various medical procedures like surgeries, dialysis, radiotherapy, day care procedures. Among national and international travellers of Ballia, 1% tested positive for COVID-19. Most COVID-19 affected area of Ballia in second wave was Hanumanganj block {Sample Positivity Rate (PR) = 7.1}, followed by Rasara (PR= 6.4), Murli Chapara (PR= 5.9), Bansdeeh (PR= 5.1), Dubahad (PR= 4.7), Ballia City (PR= 4.6), Chilkahar (PR= 4.6), Siar (PR= 4.3), Beruwarbari (PR= 4.2), Pandah (PR=4.1), Revati (PR=4.1), Nagara (PR=3.9), Maniyar (PR=3.9), Gadwar (PR=3.8), Belahari (PR= 3.1), Bairiya (PR= 2.9), Sohaon (PR= 2.9) and Nawanagar (PR= 2.2) block of Ballia district. Among total COVID-19-positive cases during the second wave, about 78% tested positive by RT-PCR Test, 21% tested positive by Rapid Antigen, and 0.8% tested positive from CB-NAAT and TrueNat (Table 3.1).

During the second wave of COVID-19, 99 reporting units were functional for testing and reporting COVID-19 cases, out of which 37% were publicly funded

Table 3.1 COVID-19 Waves Comparison

Variable	First Wave	Second Wave	Third Wwave
Duration of wave	10 May 2020 to 27 January 2021	20 March 21 to 19 June 21	31 December 21 to 18 February 22
Attack rate	0.002	0.004	0.00029
Positivity rate	3.2	4.3	0.007
Gender: Male	69%	68%	65%
Paediatric (0–15 years)	7%	6.5%	12%
Rural case	85%	93%	85%
Random sampling	42%	16%	31%
Asymptomatic contacts	27%	18%	16%
Symptomatic cases	12%	18%	3%
Field activities	17%	47%	46%
Cases for medical procedures	1%	0.7%	0.6%
Traveller tested positive	0.6%	1%	3%
Five most covid affected area	Hanumanganj (PR=7.85), Ballia City (5.58), Gadwar (3.13), Beruwarbari (3.11), Siar (3)	Hanumanganj (PR=7.1), Rasara (PR= 6.4), Murli Chapara (PR= 5.9), Bansdih (PR= 5.1), Dubahad (PR= 4.7)	Hanumanganj (PR = 1.5), Rasara (PR= 1.0), Revati (PR= 1), Nagara (PR= 1), Chilkahar (PR = 0.92)
Rapid antigen test	41%	21%	31%
RT-PCR	55%	78%	67%
CB-NAAT and TrueNat.	4%	0.8%	2%
Total reporting unit (RU)	77	99	56
Government RU	44%	37%	39%
Private RU	56%	63%	61%
Cases reported by Govt.	95%	96%	91%
Cases reported by Pvt.	5%	4%	9%
IMS-BHU (Govt.)	49%	74%	35% (BRD Gorakhpur)
Ballia Antigen Lab and District Hospital Ballia (Govt.)	41%	20% (bcz only antigen)	29% (Ballia Antigen Lab)
Heritage Hospital Varanasi	0.9%	–	–
Apex Hospital Varanasi.	0.5%	–	–
Average time for RT PCR result	1.5 days	1.6 days	Less than one day
Death	127	293	13
Death on portal	107	126	12
Death not on portal	20	167	01
CFR	13 per 1,000 people	21.7 per 1,000 people	12 per 1,000 people
Deceased	95 (75%) Male, 28 (25%) Female	200 (68%) Male, 93 (32%) Female	7 (54%) Male, 6 (46%) Female
Deceased children 0–15	03	00	03
Deceased aged >60 years	53% (68/127)	41% (119/293)	50% (6/12)

(Continued)

Table 3.1 (Continued)

Variable	First Wave	Second Wave	Third Wwave
Age-specific CFR, > 60 years	6.7 per 100 positive cases	6.7 (119/1,780) per 100 positive cases	4.3 (6/138) per 100 positive cases
Place of death	For all cases health facility	22 died in the home, 15 on the way to the hospital, 256 in hospital	02 died in the home, 02 on the way to the hospital, 09 in hospital
Home isolated	74%	96%	98.7%
Admitted in health facilities	26%	04%	1.3%

healthcare facilities (government institutions) and 63% were privately owned healthcare facilities (private institutions). Out of the total cases reported during the second wave of COVID-19, 96% were from government institutions, and 4% were from private institutions. The maximum number of COVID-19 cases (74%) were reported by the Institute of Medical Sciences (IMS), a government institution situated in Varanasi city of UP, followed by Ballia Antigen Lab (20%) and BRD Medical College Gorakhpur (4%). Most of the cases from private institutions were reported from various hospitals and laboratories running in the cities and nearby districts, i.e., Varanasi and Azamgarh. The average time taken to get the RT PCR result for a resident of Ballia during the second COVID-19 wave was 1.6 days. There was a total of 293 deaths reported during the second wave in Ballia, out of which 126 deceased cases were registered on the "upcovid19track" portal, and 167 deceased cases were reported to the district disaster cell Ballia after the announcement of compensation by the government for deaths due to COVID-19.

The key informants revealed that due to the large number of cases reported to the health facility in a shorter period, acute shortage of data entry operators and non-reporting of COVID-19 positive cases by many private health care facilities created a difficult situation updating the data of all COVID-19 positive cases on the "upcovid19track" portal. The CFR was 21.7 per 1,000 positive cases; out of the total deceased, 200 (68%) were male, and 93 (32%) were female. All reported deceased cases belong to the age group of 20 and above. Among the deceased, 41% (119) of deaths were reported among senior citizens (60 years and above) with an age-specific CFR of 6.7 per 100 positive cases and a SPR of 4.7. Among reported deceased cases, 22 died at their home, 15 on the way to the hospital, and 256 expired at various health facilities. Out of the total cases reported during the second wave, 96% were isolated at their homes, much more than in the first wave of COVID-19, and 04% were admitted to health facilities. During the second wave of COVID-19, one private healthcare facility was designated as an L2 facility for managing moderate to severe cases infected by COVID-19. For better management of COVID-19 cases in the district, 84 doctors of alternative medicine systems like Ayurveda, Yunani, and Homeopathy were pooled and trained to work in the COVID-19 rapid response team. Along with the distribution of Allopathic medicine kits to symptomatic home-isolated cases, AYUSH kits were distributed to all asymptomatic cases (UNI 2021). From 19 June 2021 onward, the number of COVID-19 cases reported in Ballia started declining in binary numbers, indicating the end of the second wave.

COVID-19: Third Wave Situational Analysis and Preparedness

After facing the two waves of the COVID-19 pandemic, it has been realised that the health infrastructure needs to be strengthened to save lives and for better clinical management of COVID-19 cases in the district; it has also been observed that paediatric age group was much less affected in the previous two waves of COVID-19 than the adult and elderly population. With support from the state government, Ballia established the "Paediatric Intensive Care Unit (PICU)" and made it functional on 27 October 2020. Also, four L1 healthcare facilities (Khejuri, Sonbarsa, Reoti, Siyar) were made functional for managing the district's mild to moderate paediatric cases. During the second wave, it was observed that the oxygen demand increased exponentially due to respiratory distress among COVID-19 patients, which caused acute shortage and crisis. Given this, the first oxygen generation plant was established in Ballina on 25 May 2021 in the district hospital. To strengthen and assess the preparedness of health care facilities and to identify the gaps, four "Mock Drills" were conducted from 27 August to 18 December 2021 in the district under the supervision of senior officials of the health department deployed from the state as nodal officers' for better management of COVID-19 cases. The COVID-19 vaccination for children aged 15–17 was also started on 03 January 2022 (Moini, 2022) and onwards in Ballia, and vaccination for 12- to 14-year-old children was started on 16 March 2022. By taking note of the lesson learned from the previous two waves of COVID-19, the booster dose of the COVID-19 vaccine for healthcare workers was started on 10 January 2022 (Arora 25 December 2021) and the booster dose for all adults above 18 years of age was started on 15 July 2022. To minimise the effect of the upcoming third wave of COVID-19, the health department decided to gear up the COVID-19 vaccination in the district. An increased trend of vaccination was noted from the date of commencement of vaccination till mid-September 2021; after that, the vaccination drive declined rapidly, and the district ranked lowest in the state; after that the district administration started daily review from 17 November 2021 onwards, which leads to an increase in Vaccination Drive exponentially, as evident from the graph (Figure 3.1).

The quality of work and daily feedback of the vaccination drive was monitored and evaluated by international agencies like World Health Organization (WHO) and United Nations Children's Fund (UNICEF). To achieve the immunisation target, the district administration has taken all the government departments on board and taken their help in mobilising beneficiaries for vaccination. The call centres were established at all the blocks and district level. Ground-level Integrated Child Development Services (ICDS) staff, Panchayati Raj Institutions (PRI) staff, Supply office, Education, and Revenue departments were deployed to mobilise beneficiaries for vaccination. Staff from PRI and health department employees were involved in feeding vaccination data on the CoWin portal. To ensure rapid immunisation, district-level officers from all the government departments were sent for supportive supervision of the field staff involved in the vaccination drive. Digital technologies like GPS cameras, Location trackers, and communication with field teams via social media were used to rectify any gaps identified during monitoring. Slow-performing cohorts and pockets were identified and strengthened at the block and district levels. Unimmunised clusters and populations were identified and targeted focused immunisation activities were conducted to vaccinate them. Vaccination teams from the health department were working biphasically (i.e., fixed session in the first half of the day till noon, then door-to-door vaccination in the second half of the day) to vaccinate the maximum number of beneficiaries in a single given day.

Daily evening review meetings were conducted by the District Magistrate (DM), Chief Development Officer (CDO) and Chief Medical Officer (CMO) of the district, and a micro-level team-based review was conducted to identify and rectify any gaps noted during the vaccination drive. Well-performing staff from various government departments who have helped in the vaccination drive were identified and felicitated by the DM. To ensure community vaccination, a survey drive was conducted from 24 to 29 January 2022 to search left-out persons for COVID-19 vaccination. The survey was initially conducted by Accredited Social Health Activists (ASHA) of the health department; subsequently, ground-level staff of other departments like ICDS and PRI were also involved in searching and reaching out to every unvaccinated individual aged 15 years and above. To strengthen the COVID-19 sampling, apart from all Lab Technicians, all the supervisory level health staff like the Health Supervisor, Community Health Officer, Pharmacists and AYUSH Medical Officers were trained (total 251) for COVID-19 sampling.

During the second wave of COVID-19, a huge demand and supply gap was noticed for the Oxygen. Given this, eight oxygen generation plants were established in the district with a capacity of 2,850 litres per minute (LPM) of oxygen supply. Additionally, 657 oxygen cylinders (B Type: 516 and D Type: 141) and 712 oxygen concentrators (5 L: 363 and 10 L: 349) were also procured from various sources.

The third wave of the SARS-CoV-2 epidemic was declared to be started on December 3 2021, in the district, during which 1,082 COVID-19-positive cases were reported in 50 days (from 31 December 2021 to 18 February 2022) with an AR of 0.00029 and SPR of 0.007. During the third wave of COVID-19, 85% of cases were reported from rural areas and 15% from urban areas of Ballia. Out of the total COVID-19 cases in the third wave, 65% were male.

Among the total cases reported, 12% belong to the paediatric age group of 0–15 years. Out of the total cases reported, most of the cases 31% were picked up on random sampling, 16% were asymptomatic contacts of COVID-19-positive persons, 3% were symptomatic cases, 46% cases were detected in various field activities like antenatal check-ups (ANC) camps, village health sanitation and nutrition days (VHSNDs). House to house campaign targeted focused sampling among various segments of society like venders, shopkeepers, school-going children,

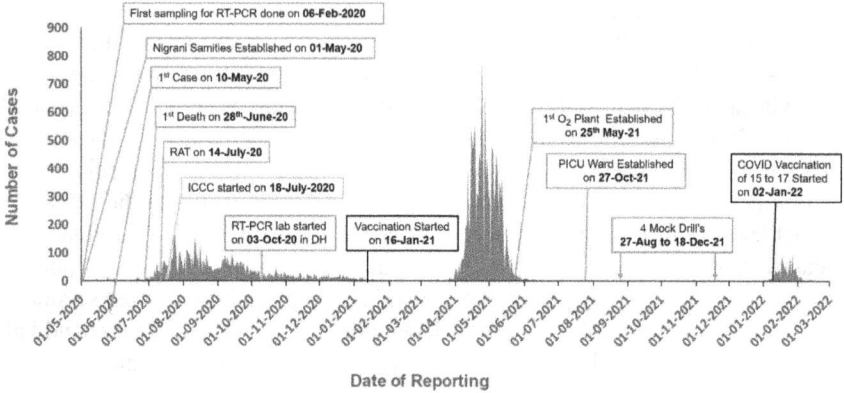

Figure 3.3 Management of COVID-19 at a Glance.

offices, bus and railway stations; 0.6% of COVID-19 cases were detected among the patients planning for various medical procedures like surgeries, dialysis, radiotherapy, day care procedures. Among national and international travellers of Ballia, 3% tested positive for COVID-19.

Most COVID-19 affected area of Ballia in third wave were Hanumanganj block (PR= 1.5), followed by Rasara (PR= 1.0), Revati (PR= 1), Nagara (PR= 1), Chilkahar (PR= 0.92), Bairiya (PR= 0.9), Pandah (PR= 0.7), Maniyar (PR= 0.7), Gadwar (PR= 0.7), Belahari (PR= 0.7), Bansdeeh (PR= 0.56), Murli Chapara (PR= 0.52), Ballia City (PR= 0.52), Sohaon (PR= 0.5), Siar (PR= 0.45), Beruwarbari (PR= 0.39), Dubahad (PR= 0.35), and Nawanagar (PR= 0.2). Among total COVID-positive cases during the third wave, 67% tested positive by RT-PCR Test, 31% tested positive by Rapid Antigen, and 2% tested positive from CB-NAAT and TrueNat. All the COVID-19 cases during the third wave in Ballia were reported from 56 Health Care Institutions, of which 39% were government institutions and 61% were private facilities. Out of the total cases, 91% were reported from government institutions, and 9% were from private institutions. Among government institutions, the maximum % of COVID-19 cases, 35%, were reported by BRD Medical College Gorakhpur, followed by Ballia Antigen Lab 29%. Most Private Institution cases were reported from various hospitals and laboratories in Varanasi and Lucknow. The average time taken to get the RT PCR result for an individual of Ballia was less than one day in the third wave of COVID-19 (Figure 3.3).

There were a total of 13 deaths reported during the third wave of COVID-19 in Ballia, with a CFR of 12 per 1,000 positive cases (Figure 3.3), with one death case reported to the administration directly during this period. Out of the total deceased, 7 were male, and 6 were female. Out of 13 deaths, nine deaths have occurred in the health facility, two deaths in the home and two deaths occurred in the ambulance during referral. Among the deceased, ten were adults, two children and one neonate. The death audit committee identified that among the deceased, 11 cases were with comorbidities like coronary artery disease, chronic renal failure, hypertension, and diabetes and the remaining two deceased had no comorbidities. It was also noted during the death audit that among the deceased, three cases were fully vaccinated with two doses of the COVID-19 vaccine, one was partially vaccinated with a single dose, and nine cases were not vaccinated for COVID-19. It was also noted that before referring the deceased to the higher health centre, out of district Ballia, eight cases visited the District Hospital Ballia, out of which six cases were not tested for COVID-19 before referral. Among the deceased, 50% of deaths were reported among senior citizens (60 years and above) with age-specific CFR of 4.3 per 100 positive cases and a SPR of 1.03. Out of the total cases reported in the third COVID-19 wave, 98.7% were isolated at home, and 1.3% were admitted to health facilities.

Discussion

In our study, we found that the Epidemic curve of the first wave of COVID-19 in district Ballia was a propagated curve, in which multiple peaks were noted in 262 days whereas the epidemic curve of the second wave was bell-shaped, in which a greater number of cases were reported in comparatively much lesser duration. The third wave of COVID-19 had a comparatively much smaller number of cases than the previous two waves with the bell-shaped epidemic curve. A similar trend of COVID-19 cases was also observed for UP (Govt. of India, 2020) and India (WHO, 2022b). We observed that the AR and SPR of COVID-19 were higher in the second wave than that of the first and third wave of COVID-19. The CFR of COVID-19 in the second wave was much higher than that of 1 and 2 waves. In the first wave of COVID-19, more than 80% of deceased cases were registered on the official portal of the UP Government; in the second wave, more than half of the death cases were not registered on the portal due to a lack of human resources for data entry and lack of reporting of all COVID-positive cases by all healthcare facilities. Most deceased cases in the third wave were registered on the portal due to fewer cases than in the previous two waves, the availability of skilled staff, and better case reporting. We observed the majority of deaths among senior citizens aged 60 years and above in all three waves of COVID-19, with a greater age-specific mortality ratio in the first two waves of COVID-19 than that of the third wave in Ballia. Various other researchers have also reported the increased mortality among the elderly population due to COVID-19 (Agrawal et al., 2021; Munayco et al., 2020). There is no death reported among children aged less than 15 years of age in the second wave, whereas in the first and third wave, three deaths were reported in this age group. During the first wave, all the deceased cases died in healthcare facilities; in the second and third waves, COVID-19 deaths were also reported in homes and transit. All the cases referred to the tertiary care units from the district hospital were not screened for COVID-19. We noted that the males were more affected by COVID-19 than the females; other researchers also recorded similar findings regarding COVID-19 (Cortis, 2020). Some researchers reported that women's movement and travel were less than men's in mid-sized cities and rural areas (Mahadevia & Advani, 2016), probably due to less exposure to the outer environment and better humoral immunity among women (Fink & Klein,

2018). We observed that the number of COVID-19 cases was higher in rural areas in the second wave as compared to the first wave of COVID-19; a similar finding was also reported by other Indian researchers (Gupta et al., 2022). We found that the number of COVID-19-positive children aged 15 years and under was two times more in the third COVID-19 wave than in the first two waves, as warned by the experts (Sitlhou, 2021; Sutaria, 2021). From the onset of the COVID-19 epidemic in Ballia, the main diagnostic modality for COVID-19 was rapid antigen test, RT-PCR, CB-NAAT, and TrueNat. More than half of the COVID-19 cases were diagnosed from RT-PCR during the first and third wave, whereas more than three-fourths of cases in the second wave were diagnosed from RT-PCR. During the first wave of COVID-19 in Ballia, most cases were diagnosed in random sampling. In contrast, most cases were identified during various field activities in the second and third waves. More than half of the healthcare facilities reporting COVID-19-positive cases during the COVID-19 pandemic were private institutions. However, as far as the number of cases is concerned, only one-tenth of these cases were reported by private institutions. Among the government institutions, most cases in the first and second waves were reported by IMS-BHU, Varanasi. In contrast, in the third wave, most cases were reported by the government medical college in Gorakhpur. We found that the average time taken to get the RT-PCR result during the first two waves of COVID-19 was more than a day, whereas, in the third wave, RT-PCR results were given to the patients on the same day of sample collection. We observed that the Hanumanganj block of Ballia was the most affected by the COVID-19 pandemic, followed by the Rasada block. In the first wave of COVID-19, around one-fourth of the cases were hospitalised; the hospitalisation rate in the second and third waves dropped drastically, and most cases were cured in home Isolation.

Test, Track, and Treat remained the main preventive strategy for COVID-19 in India (Sea & Coast, 2020; Joshi & Mehendale, 2021); because of this, since the beginning of the COVID-19 pandemic as per the directions of the state government district has also strengthened its surveillance system by establishing the Integrated Command and Control Centre which has helped in better case management and surveillance. Establishing an RT-PCR lab and dedicated COVID-19 facilities has strengthened the district's response to the COVID-19 pandemic. By the end of the first wave, COVID-19 vaccination was started in the district, but the vaccination drive gained much momentum in the second wave of COVID-19. Due to the sizeable unimmunised population, high transmissibility of the mutated virus and lack of COVID-19-appropriate behaviour (Jain et al. 2021), there was a phenomenal speed of SARS-CoV-2 in the second wave as compared to the first wave in the district. The first and second waves of COVID-19 provided ample data for preparation for the third wave; analysis of these data and learning from past experiences guided the action taken during the third wave. We observed that the peak of the third wave remained much less than that of the first and second waves. The mortality has also reduced to more than 20 times in the third wave as compared to the second wave of COVID-19 due to a massive vaccination drive leading to the immunisation of all residents of the district Ballia with the first dose of COVID-19 vaccine, training of health personnel and strengthening of the health system. Due to the decreased number of cases, the overall activities of the common people in the district remained much less affected in the third wave as compared to the first and second wave of COVID-19. Many other researchers have also observed declining COVID-19 cases after mass immunisation (Zachreson et al., 2021; De-Leon et al., 2021; Arbel et al., 2022). We conducted our study mainly based on secondary data collected and uploaded on the government-owned "http://upcovid19tracks.in" portal by many governments and private healthcare facilities, and key informant interviews; hence, along with the interviewer bias, data collection and feeding bias cannot be ruled out. To minimise data collection and feeding bias, the district surveillance unit (DSU) has trained the healthcare staff involved in COVID-19 case management, data collection and updating on the portal and was monitored by DSU daily. We recommend updating all COVID-19 cases on the government portal, focusing on the care of elderly persons, screening all patients for COVID-19 before referring them to higher treatment facilities and screening a greater number of persons for COVID-19 by private healthcare facilities. We also recommend conducting detailed statistical analyses of epidemiological and social studies in the underdeveloped districts and areas of UP and India to understand the disease progression, spread, and social impact in a better way in order to prevent such epidemics in these areas in the future.

Acknowledgement

We thank our families and friends for supporting us while preparing this manuscript.

References

Agrawal, H., Das, N., Nathani, S., Saha, S., Saini, S., Kakar, S. S., et al. (2021). An assessment on impact of COVID-19 infection in a gender-specific manner. *Stem Cell Reviews and Reports*, *17*(1), 94–112. https://doi.org/10.1007/s12015-020-10048-z.

Ambika, S., Basappa, U., Singh, A., Gonugade, V., & Tholiya, R. (2021). Impact of social lockdown due to COVID-19 on environmental and health risk indices in India. *Environmental Research*, *196*, 110932. https://doi.org/10.1016/j.envres.2021.110932.

Andersen, K. G., Rambaut, A., Lipkin, W. I., Holmes, E. C., & Garry, R. F. (2020). The proximal origin of SARS-CoV-2. *Nature Medicine*, *26*(4), 450–452. https://doi.org/10.1038/s41591-020-0820-9.

Andrews, M. A., Areekal, B., Rajesh, K. R., Krishnan, J., Suryakala, R., Krishnan. B., et al. (2020). First confirmed case of COVID-19 infection in India: A case report. *Indian Journal of Medical Research*, *151*(5), 490–492. https://doi.org/10.4103/ijmr.IJMR_2131_20.

Arbel, R., Moore, C. M., Sergienko, R., & Pliskin, J. (2022). How many lives do COVID vaccines save? Evidence from Israel. *American Journal of Infection Control, 50*(3), 258–261. https://doi.org/10.1016/j.ajic.2021.12.019.

Arora, N. (2021). India to give COVID-19 booster shots to healthcare workers from Jan. 10. *Reuters*. Retrieved October 15, 2022, from https://www.reuters.com/world/india/india-give-covid-19-booster-shots-healthcare-workers-jan-10-2021-12-25/

Ballia Population. (2021/2022). District Tehsils List, Uttar Pradesh. 11.10.2022.

Beck, U. (1992). *Risk society: Towards a new modernity*. Translated by Ritter, Mark. London: Sage Publications.

Begum, H., Neto, A. S., Alliegro, P., Broadley, T., Trapani, T., Campbell. L.T., et al. (2022). People in intensive care with COVID-19: Demographic and clinical features during the first, second, and third pandemic waves in Australia. *Medical Journal of Australia, 217*(7), 352–60. https://doi.org/10.5694/mja2.51590.

CDC. (2022). *Epi Info™*. Retrieved September 16, 2022, from https://www.cdc.gov/epiinfo/index.html

Coady, D. (2003). Conspiracy theories and official stories. *International Journal of Applied Philosophy, 17*(2), 197–209. https://doi.org/10.5840/ijap200317210.

Cortis, D. (2020). On determining the age distribution of COVID-19 pandemic. *Frontiers in Public Health*. Retrieved October 17, 2022, from https://www.frontiersin.org/articles/10.3389/fpubh.2020.00202

Coady, D. (2021). Conspiracy theory as heresy. *Educational Philosophy and Theory, 55*(7), 756–759. https://doi.org/10.1080/00131857.2021.1917364.

De-Leon, H., Calderon-Margalit. R., Pederiva, F., Ashkenazy, Y., & Gazit, D. (2021). This is the first indication of the effect of COVID-19 vaccinations on the course of the outbreak in Israel. *medRxiv*. https://doi.org/10.1101/2021.02.02.21250630.

Directorate of Medical & Health Services, Uttar Pradesh. (2022). Retrieved October 14, 2022, from https://dgmhup.gov.in/

DSO Panel. (2022). *District Surveillance Officers*. Retrieved October 11, 2022, from https://upcovid19tracks.in/admin/positive-cases

Fink, A. L., & Klein, S. L. (2018). The evolution of greater humoral immunity in females than males: Implications for vaccine efficacy. *Current Opinion in Physiology, 6*, 16–20. https://doi.org/10.1016/j.cophys.2018.03.010.

Freire, P. (1970). *Pedagogy of oppressed*. New York: Seabury Press.

Fricker, M. (2007). Epistemic Injustice. Oxford: Oxford University Press.

Giddens, A. (1991). *Modernity and self identity*. Cambridge: Polity Press.Giddens, A. (1999). Risk and responsibility. *The Modern Law Review, 62*(1), 1–10. https://doi.org/10.1111/1468-2230.00188

Govt. of India. (2020). *IndiaFightsCorona COVID-19*. March 16. MyGov.In. https://www.mygov.in/covid-19/.

Govt. of UP. (2022). *Shasanadesh*. http://shasanadesh.up.gov.in/.

Gupta, D., Biswas, D., & Kabiraj, P. (2022). COVID-19 outbreak and urban dynamics: Regional variations in India. *GeoJournal, 87*(4), 2719–2737. https://doi.org/10.1007/s10708-021-10394-6.

Jain, V. K., Iyengar, K. P., & Vaishya, R. (2021). Differences between first wave and second wave of COVID-19 in India. *Diabetes and Metabolic Syndrome: Clinical Research and Reviews, 15*(3), 1047–1048. https://doi.org/10.1016/j.dsx.2021.05.009.

James, N., Menzies, M., & Radchenko, P. (2021). COVID-19 second-wave mortality in Europe and the United States. *Chaos: An Interdisciplinary Journal of Nonlinear Science, 31*(3), 031105. https://doi.org/10.48550/arXiv.2012.13197.

Joshi, R. K., & Mehendale, S. M. (2021). Prevention and control of COVID-19 in India: Strategies and options. *Medical Journal, Armed Forces India, 77*(2), S237–S241. https://doi.org/10.1016/j.mjafi.2021.05.009.

Keeley, B. (1999). Of conspiracy theories. *The Journal of Philosophy, 96*(3), 109–126.

Koshy, J. (2021). Vaccines for all above 18 from May 1: States can buy directly. *The Hindu*, April 19, 2022. https://www.thehindu.com/news/national/from-may-1-everyone-over-18-years-eligible-for-covid-19-vaccination-government/article34359940.ece.

Lupton, D. (2016). Digital risk society. In Adam Burgess, Alberto Alemanno and Jens Zinn (eds.) *The Routledge Handbook of Risk Studies*. London: Routledge, pp. 301–309.

Machiavelli, N. (1532). *The Prince,* New Delhi: Fingerprint Classics (Reprint 2022).

Mahadevia, D., & Advani, D. (2016). Gender differentials in travel pattern – the case of a mid-sized city, Rajkot, India. *Transportation Research Part D: Transport and Environment, 44,* 292–302. https://doi.org/10.1016/j.trd.2016.01.002.

MoHFW. (2022). *Information on COVID-19 vaccines.* Retrieved October 12, 2022, from https://www.mohfw.gov.in/

Moini, M. (2022). Should you get your children vaccinated against COVID-19? *UNICEF.* Retrieved October 15, 2022, from https://www.unicef.org/india/stories/should-you-get-your-children-vaccinated-against-covid-19

Munayco, C., Chowell, G., Tariq, A., Undurraga, E. A., & Mizumoto, K. (2020). Risk of death by age and gender from CoVID-19 in Peru. *Aging (Albany, NY), 12*(14), 13869–13881.

Papa, M. J., Singhal, A., & Papa, W. H. (2006). *Organising for social change: A dialectical journey of theory and praxis.* New Delhi: Sage India Publications.

Pauly, M. (2020). Conspiracy theories. *Internet Encyclopedia of Philosophy: A Peer-Reviewed Academic Resource.* https://iep.utm.edu/conspiracy-theories/#H5.

Popper, K. R. (1966). *The open society and its enemies*: *The high tide of prophecy* (Vol. 2, 5th ed.). London: Routledge and Kegan Paul.

Popper, K. R. (1972). *Conjectures and refutations* (4th ed.). Routledge and Kegan Paul.

Prasad, R.K. Kumar, A and Srivastava, N. K. (2021). Socio-economic security of migrant workers after COVID-19: Analysis of reverse migration in Uttar Pradesh. *The Eastern Anthropologists, 74*(2), 273–295.

Sarkar, A., Chakrabarti, A. K., & Dutta, S. (2021). COVID-19 infection in India: A comparative analysis of the second wave with the first wave. *Pathogens, 10*(9), 1222. https://doi.org/10.3390/pathogens10091222.

Sea and Coast. (2020). Following the "TEST, TRACK, TREAT" strategy, India tests nearly 3.7 crore. Retrieved October 17, 2022, from https://www.seaandcoast.in/News/20663/following-%E2%80%9Ctest-track-treat%E2%80%9D-strategy-india-tests-nearly-3-7-crore

Seong, H., Hyun, H. J., Yun, J. G., Noh, J. Y., Cheong, H. J., Kim, W. J., et al. (2021). Comparison of the second and third waves of the COVID-19 pandemic in South Korea: Importance of early public health intervention. *International Journal of Infectious Diseases, 104,* 742–745. https://doi.org/10.1016/j.ijid.2021.02.004.

Sitlhou, M. (2021). Children, Covid-19, and India's looming third wave. *The BMJ, 374*(2328). https://doi.org/10.1136/bmj.n2328.

Stephanie, S., & Dylan, G. (2020). The global economic impact of COVID-19. *CSIS.* www.csis.org/analysis/global-economic-impacts-covid-19.

Strong, P. (1990). Epidemic psychology: A model. *Sociology of Health and Illness, 12*(3), 249–259. https://doi.org/10.1111/1467-9566.ep11347150.

Sutaria, S. (2021, August 23) Third COVID wave could peak in oct, and children could be at risk: Govt panel. *Boom.* Retrieved October 17, 2022, from https://www.boomlive.in/coronavirus-outbreak/india-third-covid-wave-october-children-covid-risk-ndma-govt-panel-tells-pmo-14414

UNI. (2021, May 9). *UP Govt's medicine, Ayush kits emerge as a boon in the fight against Covid-19.* Retrieved July 13, 2023, from https://www.uniindia.com/up-govt-s-medicine-ayush-kits-emerge-as-boon-in-fight-against-covid-19/north/news/2391476.html

Ward, P. R. (2020). A sociology of the Covid-19 pandemic: A commentary and research agenda for sociologists. *Journal of Sociology, 56*(4), 726–735.

WHO. (2022a). *Archived: WHO Timeline – COVID-19*. Retrieved October 11, 2022, from https://www.who.int/news/item/27-04-2020-who-timeline---covid-19

WHO. (2022b). *India: WHO coronavirus disease (COVID-19) dashboard with vaccination data*. Retrieved July 4, 2023, from https://covid19.who.int

Worldometer. (2022). *Countries where COVID-19 has spread*. Retrieved October 11, 2022, from https://www.worldometers.info/coronavirus/countries-where-coronavirus-has-spread/

Zachreson, C., Chang, S. L., Cliff, O. M., & Prokopenko, M. (2021). How will mass vaccination change COVID-19 lockdown requirements in Australia? *The Lancet Regional Health – Western Pacific*, *14*, 100224. https://doaj.org/article/43d5e28cc67a4bbe822acbd0b73624e0.

4 Speculated Anticipatory Anxiety of Social Interactions Post-COVID-19 Lockdown and the Reality Check

Sneha Mittal, Sanjay Kumar, and Vineet Gairola

Introduction

The coronavirus pandemic, commonly known as COVID-19, originated in the sea-food market of Wuhan, China (Cascella et al., 2020). Its impact quickly covered the whole world with its monstrous effect. In January 2021, initial reported deaths in various countries exhibited symptoms of a highly contagious viral illness char-acterised by severe acute respiratory concerns (Cascella et al., 2020; Singh et al., 2020). Due to the pandemic, the world witnessed more than 6.9 million deaths within three years (WHO, 2023; Cascella et al., 2020).

The cross-border transmission of the virus primarily occurred due to the active movement through airspace (Sun et al., 2020), with countries implementing lock-down measures at different times during the first trimester of 2021 (Piryani et al., 2020; Verma et al., 2020). The imposition of the lockdown was aimed at restraining the spread of the virus, which proved deadly to humans on both domestic and global levels, by abruptly restricting the population movement (Piryani et al., 2020). With the toll of impacted countries reaching above 100 by March 2020 (Verma et al., 2020) and above 213 countries by May 2020 (Piryani et al., 2020), a few countries implemented complete lockdowns while some went for partial lockdowns and a few delayed or avoided formal lockdowns, imposing limited restrictions and selec-tive quarantine (Verma et al., 2020; Oum & Wang, 2020). Countries not following strict shutdowns and allowing unnecessary services experienced a surge in con-firmed cases. Additionally, a few countries where the population did not maintain social distancing, implement lockdowns, or follow quarantine rules were penalised (Oum & Wang, 2020).

Social distancing, self-isolation, and quarantine, whether maintained voluntar-ily or due to legal obligations (Suppawittaya et al., 2020), played a crucial role in containing the more severe spread of the virus. However, these measures resulted in impacting mental health adversely, along with deteriorating physical health and an increase in confirmed cases and deaths (Pancani et al., 2021). Social isolation itself negatively impacted mental well-being, leading to feelings of loneliness, depression (Riva et al., 2017), heightened levels of anxiety, stress, insomnia, obses-sion, and compulsion (Torales et al., 2020; Mazza et al., 2020). Additionally, it was also associated with generalised anxiety disorder (GAD) (Cordaro et al., 2021),

DOI: 10.4324/9781003454984-5

psychological distress (Wang et al., 2020), a sense of horror (Zhang & Ma, 2020), and even post-traumatic stress disorder (Roy et al., 2020).

Concerns related to well-being extended beyond mental health to include aspects, such as occupation, finances, education, and even social interactions, as evidenced by changes in shopping patterns (Goolsbee & Syverson, 2021). Moreover, challenges, such as an uncomfortable study environment coupled with depression, anxiety, and poor internet connectivity were observed among students of higher education (Kapasia et al., 2020; Bonal & González, 2020). The impact on the economy was evident in reduced economic activities (Singh & Ranjith, 2021), manufacturing disruptions, and disturbances in the demand and supply chain (Joshi et al., 2020), leading to labour losses (Vyas, 2020), travel restrictions (Dube-Xaba, 2021), and changes in travel pattern (Meena, 2020; Shibayama et al., 2021; Singh et al., 2022), further contributing to the complicated scenario.

The prevailing unease gave way to negative anticipation of anxiety, including concerns related to travel (Singh et al., 2022), health, finances, employment (Joshi et al., 2020), education, fear of loss of loved ones, and the restriction of personal or social freedom. This negative anticipation also involved being confined in one place and facing a survival crisis due to trouble arranging food and shelter (Onyeaka et al., 2021). Several studies affirm that the fear of contracting COVID-19 affected individuals across age groups and various roles, including health workers, mental health professionals, government officials, police, the elderly, the young, and children (Amin, 2020; Sharma et al., 2020). The widespread increase in mental stress and panic holds significant psychological implications and can potentially lead to severe mental health issues (Mohammadpour et al., 2020).

Significant differences were found in the level of fear among females as compared to males, married as compared to unmarried individuals, and people with lower levels of formal education in Cuba (Broche-Pérez et al., 2022), India (Doshi et al., 2021), and Bangladesh (Hossain et al., 2020). Notably, individuals with a psychiatric history experienced a considerable decline in mental health due to the weakening of the immune system, rendering them more susceptible to psychological (Mazza et al., 2020). The global suicide rate increased significantly during the coronavirus era (Dsouza et al., 2020; Devitt, 2020; Goyal et al., 2020; McIntyre & Lee, 2020). Nevertheless, adhering to a holistic and positive daily routine was suggested to alleviate stress (Sharma et al., 2020), while increased awareness of managing COVID-19 was found helpful (Agarwal et al., 2020).

The progression of the COVID-19 situation unfolded in various stages, involving the emergence of different variants at different times, each with its unique consequences. Ultimately, the World Health Organization (WHO) officially declared the end of the COVID-19 pandemic on 5 May 2023 (Sarker et al., 2023). The highest death count was found to be present until March 2022, touching 7 million deaths by May 2023 (WHO, 2023). The pandemic gave rise to changes in behaviour patterns in many forms, such as a reduction in the inclination to travel (Luo & Lam, 2020), an increase in anxiety related to future career prospects (Mahmud et al., 2020), and consistent handwashing, persistent fear, and a heightened sense of the need for precautions (Mohammadpour et al., 2020).

Additionally, in foreign trip planning, it was found that people had cancelled booked tickets for trains and domestic and international flights as a precautionary measure during the COVID-19 scenario (Meena, 2020).

Among the Indian population, a substantial proportion possessed a moderate to sufficient level of knowledge regarding COVID-19 infection and its preventive measures, with 72% of the surveyed population expressing support for using gloves and sanitisers (Roy et al., 2020). Social distancing and regulations mandating regular handwashing were legally imposed during the initial months of the outbreak. However, it was hypothesised that gradually, people might continue to adhere to these restrictions, thereby influencing long-established patterns of interaction and lifestyle.

The above reviews and studies demonstrate the profound impact of the COVID-19 pandemic on various aspects of life, including health, mental well-being, social behaviour, and the economy. However, there is a notable absence of exploring the impact of fear on a person's current perception of the scenarios that may prevail later. The observed changes are attributed to the current apprehension regarding future behaviour. This research aims to examine the effect of the current circumstances on subsequent behaviour and adjustment patterns. This survey research studies the levels of anticipatory anxiety among people, persisting even after the conclusion of the COVID-19 era, and assesses the dynamics of fear along with alterations in their physical and interpersonal way of being.

Material and Method

A survey was conducted by circulating a Google form containing a self-constructed questionnaire. The survey was primarily distributed through social media platforms, such as WhatsApp and Facebook and personal follow-ups. There were no exclusion criteria, and the informed consent was included in the Google form, ensuring that only individuals consenting to participate could complete the survey. The questionnaire included a short consent form and socio-demographic profile capturing information, such as age, gender, qualification, and profession. Additionally, it included 12 statements with a 5-point Likert-type statement ranging from "Absolutely," "Probably," "Not Sure," "Probably Not," and "Never." These statements were framed to gather raw information regarding the sudden behavioural changes and stress level due to the lockdown, potential ongoing changes post-lockdown, and perceived life risks. The questionnaire was not standardised due to time constraints, as standardisation would have delayed data collection beyond the initial stress period of the imposed lockdown. From August 2020 to September 2020, 409 responses were collected using snowballing. The responses received were from various states of India, including Haryana, New Delhi, Punjab, West Bengal, Assam, Kerala, Orissa, and Tamil Nadu. The responding sample was a social media and gadget-friendly population, making the response collection possible during the lockdown.

Out of 12 statements in the survey, the initial three focused on behavioural domains related to participation in outdoor activities, visits, and public interactions. The objective was to examine an individual's openness post-lockdown and assess

Table 4.1 Nature and Scoring of Question Statements

S. No.	Statement	Scoring
1	Are you worried about the uncertainty of the future? Is it academic, familial, or professional life?	Positive
2	Are you anxious about getting optimum treatment for coronavirus if it is found positive?	Positive
3	Are you scared of getting coronavirus?	Positive
4	Will you participate in religious events?	Negative
5	Will you continue cleaning and sanitising every item in your home?	Positive
6	Would you host your overseas relative or friend in your home?	Negative
7	Will you use public transport even in a rush?	Negative
8	Will you keep using masks as your routine dress-up?	Positive
9	Will you keep maintaining social distancing?	Positive

the impact of the current scenario, marked by fear and a high death toll caused by social interaction, on future perceptions of social interactions. These statements were presented in a checkbox format. The subsequent nine statements intend to measure the level of anticipatory anxiety regarding the potential exposure to COVID-19 even after the lockdown. Descriptive statistics were employed for analysis, utilising SPSS.

Scoring

The survey form was not a standardised tool. The scoring was done to categorise the raw scores into meaningful interpretations. The 12 statements included both negative and positive statements. This scoring format was based on the level of intensity of anxiety that the options showed, as demonstrated by Table 4.1.

The higher the level of anxiety, the higher the corresponding score. Negative statements were assigned scores ranging from 1 to 5 for options "Absolutely," "Probably," "Not Sure," "Probably Not," and "Never," respectively. Conversely, positive statements received scores of 5, 4, 3, 2, and 1 for the same options. This scoring system yields a minimum score of 9 and a maximum score of 45. The maximum score is equally divided into three categories, namely, low anticipation of getting infected (scores 9–21), moderate anticipation of getting infected (scores 22–33), and high anticipation of getting infected (scores 34–45).

Results

The results are divided into two sections. The first part includes the survey's descriptive results, while the second part delves into the reality check of the current scenario amid post-lockdown. The "reality check' discusses the actual application and accuracy of the anticipation anxiety that the sample perceived during the peak pandemic lockdown during the first trimester of 2020, as stated in responses to the survey.

Socio-demographic Findings

Table 4.2 provides an intricate overview of the sample's demographic composition in age, gender, qualification, and profession. As the study involved no particular

Table 4.2 Socio-Demography of the Study Sample

Variable		Frequency (N=409)	Percentage	Mean	SD
Age	13–22	140	34.2	25.24	6.860
	23–32	229	55.9		
	33–42	28	6.8		
	43–52	7	1.7		
	53–65	5	1.2		
Gender	Male	156	38	1.68	1.34
	Female	253	62		
Qualification	Matriculate	26	6.4	3.48	1.581
	Intermediate	42	10.3		
	Graduate	115	28.1		
	Postgraduate	201	49.1		
	Doctorates	14	3.4		
	M.Phil.	5	1.2		
	Diploma	4	1		
	Researchers	2	0.4		
Profession	Government job	36	8.8	6.13	2.232
	Business/entrepreneur	12	2.9		
	Academician	32	7.8		
	Medical professional	14	3.4		
	Labour	3	0.7		
	Student	298	72.9		
	Skill artisan	7	1.7		
	Homemaker	7	1.7		

inclusion criteria, the sample exhibited diversity in educational and professional backgrounds. The sample's age range ranged from 13 to 65 years, with maximum participation of young adults aged 23–32. In the age distribution, female participation was almost double that of male participation. In the qualification distribution, almost half of the participants were postgraduates, followed by graduates. Lastly, in the profession description, 70% of the sample were students, followed by government employees and academicians (Figures 4.1–4.4).

Apart from the socio-demographic data, three statements focused on the population's post-lockdown meeting preferences, preferred mode of social interaction, and the probability of planning a national or an international trip immediately after or within the upcoming six months or a year after the upliftment of the lockdown.

Everyday Interactions and Future Prospects

Table 4.3 shows the characterisation of the responses to the qualitative statements aiming to unveil the behavioural and emotional front of the population towards COVID-19 during its peak months in the year 2020. The question regarding preferences for social interactions and physical contact reveals that approximately 60% of the population favoured verbal greetings. Following this, the preference was for shaking hands only if sanitised, with hugging being the

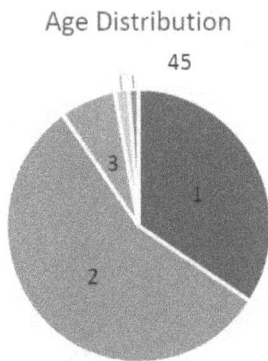

Figure 4.1 Description of Sample Age Distribution.

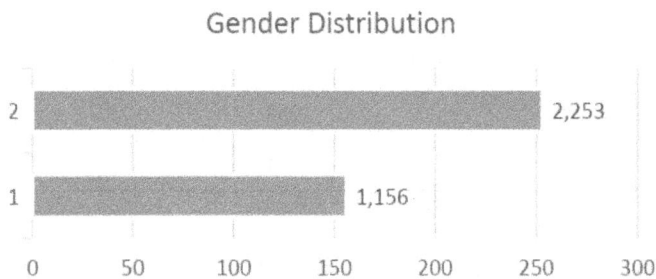

Figure 4.2 Description of Gender Distribution.

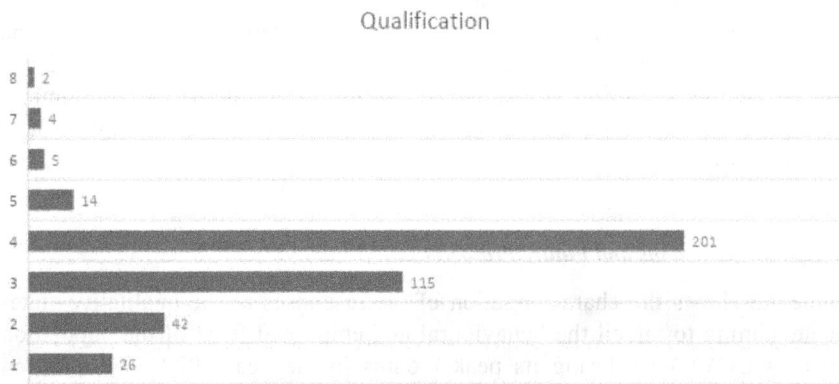

Figure 4.3 Description of Sample Qualification.

Profession

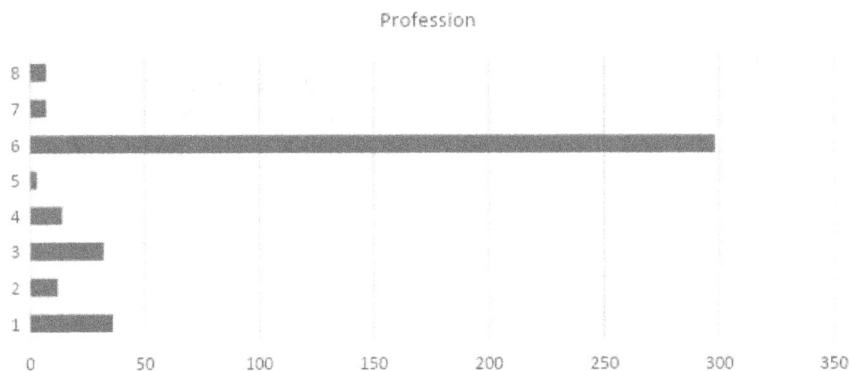

Figure 4.4 Description of Sample Profession.

Table 4.3 Frequency Distribution of Qualitative Statement Responses

Variable	Response Options	Frequency (N=409)	Percentage
When meeting someone, what would you prefer to	Greet verbally	253	61.9
	Shake hands	44	10.8
	First, sanitise, then shake hands	79	19.3
	Hug	33	8.1
	First, enquire about the pandemic history, then shake hands	40	9.8
Would you like to participate in	Hobby classes	208	50.9
	Get-together parties	141	34.5
	Hotels	48	11.7
	Pub/clubs	14	3.4
	Gyms	79	19.3
How would you plan a trip	International trip within six months	22	5.4
	International trip within one year	31	7.6
	National trip within six months	130	31.8
	National trip within one year	183	44.7
	Plan trip immediately	73	17.8

least favoured option. Individuals commonly exchange hugs or handshakes in India, particularly in non-professional settings. The shift in behaviour, driven by the fear of contamination, underscores the profound impact of fear on daily routines.

In the statement regarding participation in any public event or public space, the preference was highest towards engaging in hobby classes, while the least favoured option was attending pubs or clubs. Hotels and gyms ranked higher, followed by get-together parties. This suggests a reluctance to interact with unfamiliar individuals. Opting for hobby classes instead of evening parties is seen as more productive for self-development, justifying the fear. Furthermore, activities like hobby classes or getting together with family and friends reduce stress and increase coping ability. The third statement concerns planning and preference for future national or international trips.

Interestingly, only 17% of the sample population planned to have a trip immediately after the removal of the lockdown, though the reason needed to be assessed. The highest vote-grossing option was a national trip within one year at 44%,

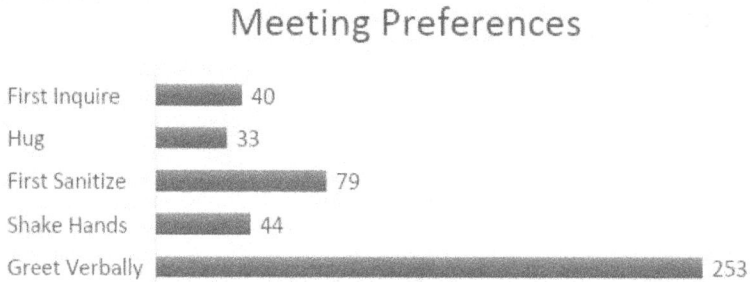

Meeting Preferences

First Inquire	40
Hug	33
First Sanitize	79
Shake Hands	44
Greet Verbally	253

Figure 4.5 Distribution of Meeting Preferences Among the Sample Post-Lockdown.

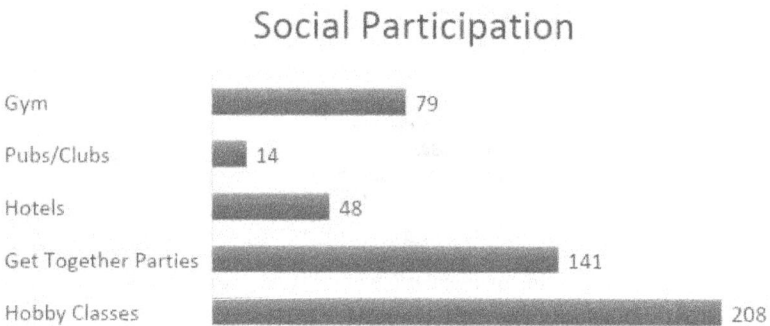

Social Participation

Gym	79
Pubs/Clubs	14
Hotels	48
Get Together Parties	141
Hobby Classes	208

Figure 4.6 Distribution of Social Participation Among the Sample Post-Lockdown.

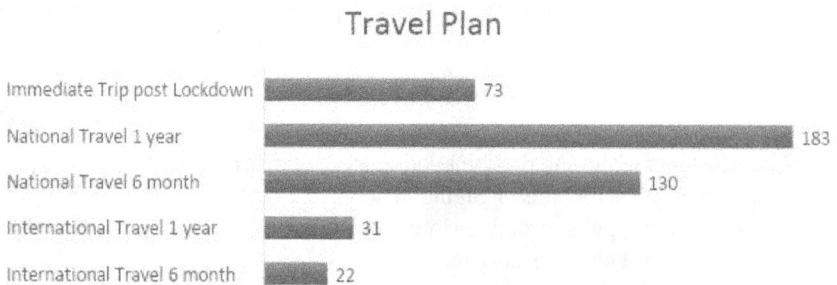

Travel Plan

Immediate Trip post Lockdown	73
National Travel 1 year	183
National Travel 6 month	130
International Travel 1 year	31
International Travel 6 month	22

Figure 4.7 Distribution of Travel Plan Among the Sample Post-Lockdown.

followed by 31% planning a national trip within six months. This indicates a preference for a one-year gap over six months when considering a domestic trip. Similarly, a one-year interval was more preferred for international trips than a six-month one (Figures 4.5–4.7).

The following nine questionnaire statements aiming to assess the anticipation regarding cognitive and behaviour patterns have been described in the number of responses and mean and SD.

4.4 Frequency Description of Responses to the Statements

In Table 4.4, the qualitative analysis of the survey questions revealed a high level of anticipation in both cognitive and behavioural aspects. Statements like "Are you worried about future uncertainty in life? Be it academic, familial, or professional life?" "Are you anxious about getting optimum treatment for Coronavirus if found Positive?" and "Are you scared of getting Coronavirus" yielded responses indicating high anxiety in a major part of responses ($n=172$), ($n=153$), and ($n=105$), respectively. Furthermore, a mixed response was found in the statement regarding the fear of getting infected by a coronavirus, as 23.5% of the sample equally responded to options, such as "Never" and "Probably." It suggests that while the population is not afraid of the virus, they nevertheless implement preventive measures, such as practising social distancing, wearing masks, using sanitisers, and preparing for potential future uncertainties.

The statements infer behavioural aspects like "Will you participate in religious events?" "Will you continue using masks, cleaning and sanitising, use public transport even in a rush and maintain social distancing?" scored the highest frequency in the "Never" option with ($n=110$), ($n=237$), ($n=227$), ($n=145$), and ($n=267$), respectively. However, the survey also indicated that people chose "probably" as an option concerning hosting their visiting overseas relatives, with ($n=102$) at the highest possibility. The quantitative findings reveal a high level of anticipatory anxiety prevailing in the sample population. High anxiety regarding coronavirus post-lockdown was found among 46.9% ($n=192$) of the sample under study, while 46.4% ($n=190$) of the population was moderately anxious. Only 6.6% ($n=27$) of the population was less anxious regarding coronavirus post-lockdown.

The second section of the analysis focuses on the "reality check" of said preferences post-lockdown. The survey was conducted, revealing a high level of prevailing anxiety among the population during the peak period. This indicates that heightened anticipation correspondingly leads to increased alterations in behaviour and cognition.

The "reality check" is done in three aspects: how people meet and greet, social interactions, and the changes in travel patterns.

After the upliftment of the lockdown, social interaction has gradually increased, although not returning to the same normalcy as before (Tang, 2021). The support and care from friends and families have increased (Zhang & Ma, 2020) along with positive mental health-related lifestyle changes (Lau et al., 2006). Adherence to safety measures has become more prevalent compared to the

Table 4.4 Frequency Description of Responses to the Statements

S. No.	Positive Statements	Absolutely	Probably	Not Sure	Probably Not	Never	Mean	SD
1	Are you worried about the uncertainty of the future? Is it academic, familial, or professional life?	172	105	61	40	31	3.848	1.27
2	Are you anxious about getting optimum treatment for coronavirus if it is found positive?	153	71	69	48	68	3.471	1.49
3	Are you scared of getting coronavirus?	105	96	50	62	96	3.127	1.52
4	Will you continue cleaning and sanitising every item in your home?	227	106	33	29	14	4.229	1.08
5w	Will you keep using masks as your routine dress-up?	237	85	40	28	19	4.205	1.15
6	Will you keep maintaining social distancing?	267	82	32	21	7	4.420	0.95

S. No.	Negative Statements	Absolutely	Probably	Not Sure	Probably Not	Never	Mean	SD
7	Will you participate in religious events?	64	90	69	76	110	3.190	1.43
8	Would you host your overseas relative or friend in your home?	98	102	94	69	46	2.665	1.30
9	Will you use public transport even in a rush?	47	58	71	88	145	3.552	1.38

pre-COVID-19 era. Safety practices during shopping, such as hygiene maintenance, observing physical distancing norms, using face masks, and using sanitisers, have become standard requirements (Sehgal et al., 2023). These observations align with survey responses indicating a continued commitment to safety measures post-lockdown. In terms of travel patterns, travel by air and travel through train reservations could be tracked more precisely than the non-reserved or general quota travelling by busses and the general coaches of trains. The travel preference reported in the survey was checked using data available on government websites and articles.

As per the records, after the sudden cessation of all public facilities to and from the entire nation on 15 March 2020, the Indian railways opened only a few trains to move migrant labourers to their home states on 21 May 2020. Gradually, only partial facilities were opened for the passengers travelling in those trains during the lockdown. It has been clearly stated that the travel behaviours within the population fluctuated during the later waves of the COVID-19 pandemic. The start of the waves was followed by a decrease in travel, while the downfall of later COVID-19 waves automatically increased the size of the travelling population (Thakur, 2022). As per the data of India Revenue Passenger Kilometres, the record low revenue of all time was seen in the year 2021, which was a drop from INR 506,690.00 in the year 2020 to INR 152,484.00 in the year 2021 (India Revenue Passengers Kilometres, 2022). Similar to the railway and bus transport facility, the services of aviation sector was also kept no to minimum for the safety and security of the passengers. Only domestic airlines were resumed by the Indian Government, a move not fully supported by the state governments, prioritising public health. However, to ensure the survival of the Indian aviation sector, a few steps were taken. In the summer of 2020, only 33% of domestic flights were scheduled, gradually increasing by September of the same year (Mallapur, 2020). Government regulations predominantly governed public air travel, yet by September 2021, approximately 13 countries had opened their doors to Indian travellers. From March 2020 to September 2021, this period amounted to about 1.5 years of restricted international travel, with destinations, such as Thailand, Maldives, Switzerland, UAE, Turkey, and Nepal allowing Indian visitors (Mallapur, 2020). While the current Indian aviation scenario has a much better traveller count, the above data shows that the trips planned by the people were curtailed in both domestic and international contexts but finally resulted in reduced travel immediately after the fall of the COVID-19 lockdown.

The respondents indicated that they anticipated they would continue to make less use of buses and trains at the end of the pandemic (Downey et al., 2022). As per the perceived anticipation during peak lockdown about the post-lockdown era, the population opted more for a personal mode of transport than public ones and other shared modes of travel like booking cabs (Meena, 2020). Additionally, Meena (2020) observed a shift towards minimising non-essential trips and a preference for healthier modes of travel, such as walking and cycling. These evolving preferences suggest a lasting impact on transportation choices, emphasising a continued emphasis on individual modes and sustainable alternatives to a greater extent even beyond the pandemic.

Conclusion

The study aimed to assess the level of anticipatory anxiety surrounding COVID-19 during the initial months of the outbreak and the implementation of lockdown measures. The results showed that personal safety measures, restricted socialising, self-permitted physical interactions, interpersonal relationships, and future uncertainties regarding health and career remained high. The findings revealed a high level of anticipatory anxiety regarding COVID-19 infection during the initial months, and this anxiety, along with feelings of insecurity, was expected to persist, potentially influencing interaction styles and travel preferences until the situation stabilises. These changes encompassed behavioural aspects (such as dressing, domestic or international travel, socialising, greeting, and hosting) and cognitive aspects (concerns about future uncertainty, treatment anxiety, and fear of viral infection). Significant behaviour and travel pattern shifts were observed before and during the lockdown. Although there was a limited intention to travel freely post-lockdown, the subsequent easing of restrictions did not necessarily reflect similar conditions. The population exhibited a higher degree of caution compared to the earlier phase. Additionally, numerous communication and interaction techniques emerged and became commonplace, including a move towards cashless transactions and online meetings. Despite these changes, psychological support and maintenance must be provided to the individuals who have recovered from COVID-19, as well as their family members, health workers, and common people, to ensure their well-being in the years to come in this ever-changing world.

Limitations and Future Suggestions

A standardised tool was not available. Hence, a survey study was designed. The study was conducted from August to October 2020, capturing a specific time frame during the pandemic. As the situation evolved rapidly, the findings may not fully represent the prolonged and dynamic nature of the crisis, limiting the generalisability of the results. The age distribution in the survey was not uniform, owing to the snowballing approach used in data collection. Future work combining survey data with qualitative methods, such as interviews or focus groups, would result in a richer understanding of individuals' experiences and perspectives, enhancing the findings' depth and validity. Additionally, diversifying the sample by including participants from various geographic locations, socio-economic backgrounds, and cultural contexts would increase the representativeness of the population under study. Furthermore, a study focused on the effectiveness of intervention strategies aimed at mitigating anticipatory anxiety and improving mental health during and after a crisis could be conducted. This could inform practical measures for future pandemics or similar events.

Acknowledgement

The authors acknowledge all the participants of the research.

References

Agarwal, V., Sharma, S., Gupta, L., Misra, D. P., Davalbhakta, S., Agarwal, V., Goel, A., & Aggarwal, S. (2020). COVID-19 and psychological disaster preparedness – an unmet need. *Disaster Medicine and Public Health Preparedness, 14*(3), 387–390.
Amin, S. (2020). The psychology of coronavirus fear: Are healthcare professionals suffering from corona-phobia? *International Journal of Healthcare Management, 13*(3), 249–256. https://doi.org/10.1080/20479700.2020.1765119
Bonal, X., & González, S. (2020). The impact of lockdown on the learning gap: family and school divisions in times of crisis. *International Review of Education, 66*(5–6), 635–655. https://doi.org/10.1007/s11159-020-09860-z

Broche-Pérez, Y., Fernández-Fleites, Z., Jiménez-Puig, E., Fernández-Castillo, E., & Rodríguez-Martin, B. C. (2022). Gender and fear of COVID-19 in a Cuban population sample. *International Journal of Mental Health and Addiction, 20,* 83–91. https://doi.org/10.1007/s11469-020-00343-8

Cascella, M., Rajnik, M., Cuomo, A., Dulebohn, S. C., & Napoli, R. D. (2020). Features, evaluation, and treatment of coronavirus (COVID-19). In: *StatPearls.* Treasure Island, FL: StatPearls Publishing.

Cordaro, M., Grigsby, T. J., Howard, J. T., Deason, R. G., Haskard-Zolnierek, K., & Howard, K. (2021). Pandemic-specific factors related to Generalized Anxiety Disorder during the initial COVID-19 protocols in the United States. *Issues in Mental Health Nursing, 42*(8), 747–757. https://doi.org/10.1080/01612840.2020.1867675

Devitt, P. (2020). Can we expect an increased suicide rate due to Covid-19? *Irish Journal of Psychological Medicine, 37*(4), 264–268. https://doi.org/10.1017/ipm.2020.46

Doshi, D., Karunakar, P., Sukhabogi, J. R., Prasanna, J. S., & Mahajan, S. V. (2021). Assessing coronavirus fear in Indian population using the fear of COVID-19 scale. *International Journal of Mental Health and Addiction, 19,* 2383–2391. https://doi.org/10.1007/s11469-020-00332-x

Downey, L., Fonzone, A., Fountas, G., & Semple, T. (2022). Impact of COVID-19 on future public transport use in Scotland. *Transportation Research Part A: Policy and Practice, 163,* 338–352. https://doi.org/10.1016/j.tra.2022.06.005

Dsouza, D. D., Quadros, S., Hyderabadwala, Z. J., & Mamun, M. A. (2020). Aggregated COVID-19 suicide incidences in India: Fear of COVID-19 infection is the prominent causative factor. *Psychiatry Research, 290,* 113145. https://doi.org/10.1016/j.psychres.2020.113145

Dube-Xaba, Z. (2021). COVID-19 lockdown and visiting friends and relatives travellers: Impact and opportunities. *African Journal of Hospitality, Tourism and Leisure, 10*(3), 856–862. https://doi.org/10.46222/ajhtl.19770720-136

Goolsbee, A., & Syverson, C. (2021). Fear, lockdown, and diversion: Comparing drivers of pandemic economic decline 2020. *Journal of Public Economics, 193,* 104311. https://doi.org/10.1016/j.jpubeco.2020.104311

Goyal, K., Chauhan, P., Chhikara, K., Gupta, P., & Singh, M. P. (2020). Fear of COVID 2019: First suicidal case in India! *Asian Journal of Psychiatry, 49,* 101989. https://doi.org/10.1016/j.ajp.2020.101989

Hossain, M. A., Jahid, M. I. K., Hossain, K. M. A., Walton, L. M., Uddin, Z., Haque, M. O., et al. (2020). Knowledge, attitudes, and fear of COVID-19 during the Rapid Rise Period in Bangladesh. *PLoS One, 15*(9), e0239646. https://doi.org/10.1371/journal.pone.0239646

India Revenue Passengers Kilometers. (2022). *India Railway: Revenue and expenditure.* Retrieved November 10, 2023, from https://www.ceicdata.com/en/india/railway-revenue-and-expenditure/revenue-passenger-kilometres

Joshi, A., Bhaskar, P., & Gupta, P. K. (2020). Indian economy amid COVID-19 lockdown: A perspective. *Journal of Pure and Applied Microbiology, 14,* 957–961. https://doi.org/10.22207/JPAM.14.SPL1.33

Kapasia, N., Paul, P., Roy, A., Saha, J., Zaveri, A., Mallick, R., et al. (2020). Impact of lockdown on learning status of undergraduate and postgraduate students during COVID-19 pandemic in West Bengal, India. *Children and Youth Services Review, 116,* 105194. https://doi.org/10.1016/j.childyouth.2020.105194

Lau, J. T., Yang, X., Tsui, H. Y., Pang, E., & Wing, Y. K. (2006). Positive mental health-related impacts of the SARS epidemic on the general public in Hong Kong and their associations with other negative impacts. *Journal of Infection, 53*(2), 114–124. https://doi.org/10.1016/j.jinf.2005.10.019

Luo, J. M., & Lam, C. F. (2020). Travel anxiety, risk attitude and travel intentions towards "travel bubble" destinations in Hong Kong: Effect of the fear of COVID-19. *International Journal of Environmental Research and Public Health, 17*(21), 7859. https://doi.org/10.3390/ijerph17217859

Mahmud, M. S., Talukder, M. U., & Rahman, S. M. (2020). Does 'Fear of COVID-19' trigger future career anxiety? An empirical investigation considering depression from COVID-19 as a mediator. *The International Journal of Social Psychiatry, 67*(1), 35–45. https://doi.org/10.1177/0020764020935488

Mallapur, C. (2020). *How COVID-19 hurt the Indian aviation industry.* Retrieved November 10, 2023, from https://www.moneycontrol.com/news/business/economy/heres-how-covid-19-has-hurt-the-indian-aviation-industry-5965511.html

Mazza, M. G., De Lorenzo, R., Conte, C., Poletti, S., Vai, B., Bollettini, I., et al. (2020). Anxiety and depression in COVID-19 survivors: Role of inflammatory and clinical predictors. *Brain, Behavior, and Immunity, 89*, 594–600. https://doi.org/10.1016/j.bbi.2020.07.037

McIntyre, R. S., & Lee, Y. (2020). Preventing suicide in the context of the COVID-19 pandemic. *World Psychiatry, 19*(2), 250–251. https://doi.org/10.1002/wps.20767

Meena, S. (2020). Impact of novel Coronavirus (COVID-19) pandemic on travel pattern: A case study of India. *Indian Journal of Science and Technology, 13*(24), 2491–2501. https://doi.org/10.17485/IJST/v13i24.958

Mohammadpour, M., Ghorbani, V., Khoramnia, S., Ahmadi, S. M., Ghvami, M., & Maleki, M. (2020). Anxiety, self-compassion, gender differences and COVID-19: Predicting self-care behaviours and fear of COVID-19 based on anxiety and self-compassion with an emphasis on gender differences. *Iranian Journal of Psychiatry, 15*(3), 213–219. https://doi.org/10.18502/ijps.v15i3.3813

Onyeaka, H., Anumudu, C. K., Al-Sharify, Z. T., Egele-Godswill, E., & Mbaegbu, P. (2021). COVID-19 pandemic: A review of the global lockdown and its far-reaching effects. *Science Progress, 104*(2), 00368504211019854. https://doi.org/10.1177/00368504211019854

Oum, T. H., & Wang, K. (2020). Socially optimal lockdown and travel restrictions for fighting communicable virus including COVID-19. *Transport Policy, 96*, 94–100. https://doi.org/10.1016/j.tranpol.2020.07.003

Pancani, L., Marinucci, M., Aureli, N., & Riva, P. (2021). Forced social isolation and mental health: a study on 1,006 Italians under COVID-19 lockdown. *Frontiers in Psychology, 12*, 663799. https://doi.org/10.3389/fpsyg.2021.663799

Piryani, R. M., Piryani, S., Piryani, S., Shakya, D. R., & Huq, M. (2020). COVID-19 and lockdown: Be logical in relaxing it. *Journal of Lumbini Medical College, 8*(1), 150–153. https://doi.org/10.22502/jlmc.v8i1.361

Riva, P., Montali, L., Wirth, J. H., Curioni, S., & Williams, K. D. (2017). Chronic social exclusion and evidence for the resignation stage: an empirical investigation. *Journal of Social and Personal Relationships, 34*(4), 541–564. https://doi.org/10.1177/0265407516644348

Roy, D., Tripathy, S., Kar, S. K., Sharma, N., Verma, S. K., & Kaushal, V. (2020). Study of knowledge, attitude, anxiety & perceived mental healthcare need in Indian population during COVID-19 pandemic. *Asian Journal of Psychiatry, 51*, 102083. https://doi.org/10.1016/j.ajp.2020.102083

Sarker, R., Roknuzzaman, A. S. M., Nazmunnahar, Shahriar, M., Hossain, M. J., & Islam, M. R. (2023). The WHO has declared the end of pandemic phase of COVID-19: Way to come back in the normal life. *Health Science Reports, 6*(9), e1544. https://doi.org/10.1002/hsr2.1544

Sehgal, R., Khanna, P., Malviya, M., & Dubey, A. M. (2023). Shopping safety practices mutate consumer buying behaviour during COVID-19 pandemic. *Vision: The Journal of Business Perspective, 27*(5), 604–615. https://doi.org/10.1177/09722629211010

Sharma, S., Kundu, A., Basu, S., Shetti, N. P., & Aminabhavi, T. M. (2020). Indians vs. COVID-19: The scenario of mental health. *Sensors International, 1*, 100038. https://doi. org/10.1016/j.sintl.2020.100038

Shibayama, T., Sandholzer, F., Laa, B., & Brezina, T. (2021). Impact of COVID-19 lockdown on commuting: A multi-country perspective. *European Journal of Transport and Infrastructure Research, 21*(1), 70–93

Singh, A. K., Agrawal, B., Sharma, A., & Sharma, P. (2020). COVID-19: Assessment of knowledge and awareness in Indian society. *Journal of Public Affairs, 20*(4), e2354. https://doi.org/10.1002/pa.2354

Singh, S., & Ranjith, M. (2021). Lockdown and its impact on education, environment and economy. *Journal of Advances in Education and Philosophy, 5*(4), 116–119.

Singh, V., Gupta, K., Agarwal, A., & Chakrabarty, N. (2022). Psychological impacts on the travel behaviour post Covid-19. *Asian Transport Studies, 8*, 100087.

Sun, X., Wandelt, S., & Zhang, A. (2020). How did COVID-19 impact air transportation? A first peek through the lens of complex networks. *Journal of Air Transport Management, 89*, 101928.

Suppawittaya, P., Yiemphat, P., & Yasri, P. (2020). Effects of social distancing, self-quarantine and self-isolation during the COVID-19 pandemic on people's well-being, and how to cope with it. *International Journal of Science and Healthcare Research, 5*(2), 12–20.

Tang, K. H. D. (2021). Controversies of the post-lockdown new normal-it may not be entirely normal. *Current Research Journal of Social Sciences & Humanities, 4*(1), 7. https://doi. org/10.12944/CRJSSH.4.1.02

Thakur, N. (2022). *2 years after lockdown: How life around India rail is slowly back on track.* Retrieved November 10, 2023, from, https://www.moneycontrol.com

Torales, J., O'Higgins, M., Castaldelli-Maia, J. M., & Ventriglio, A. (2020). The outbreak of COVID-19 coronavirus and its impact on global mental health. *International Journal of Social Psychiatry, 66*(4), 317–320. https://doi.org/10.1177/0020764020915212

Verma, B. K., Verma, M., Verma, V. K., Abdullah, R. B., Nath, D. C., Khan, H. T., Verma, A., Vishwakarma, R. K., & Verma, V. (2020). Global lockdown: An effective safeguard in responding to the threat of COVID-19. *Journal of Evaluation in Clinical Practice, 26*(6), 1592–1598.

Vyas, M. (2020). Impact of lockdown on labour in India. *The Indian Journal of Labour Economics, 63*(Suppl 1), 73–77.

Wang, H., Qian, X., Xiong, Z., Li, Z., Xiang, W., Yuan, Y., et al. (2020). The psychological distress and coping styles in the early stages of the 2019 coronavirus disease (COVID-19) epidemic in the general mainland Chinese population: A web-based survey. *PLoS One, 15*, e0233410. https://doi.org/10.1371/journal.pone.0233410

World Health Organization (WHO). (2023). *WHO coronavirus (COVID-19) dashboard.* World Health Organization. Retrieved December 10, 2023, from https://covid19.who.int/

Zhang, Y., & Ma, Z. F. (2020). Impact of the COVID-19 pandemic on mental health and quality of life among local residents in Liaoning province, China: A cross-sectional study. *International Journal of Environmental Research and Public Health, 17*(7), 2381. https://doi.org/10.3390/ijerph17072381

Appendix 1

Anticipatory Anxiety after Lockdown (Survey Form)

(All questions were marked mandatory except Name in Google Form)

1 Name _____
2 Age _____
3 Gender: a) Male _____ b) Female _____
4 Qualification:

   a Metric
   b Intermediate
   c Graduate
   d Postgraduate
   e Doctorate

5 Profession:

   a Government Job
   b Business/Entrepreneur
   c Bank
   d Academician
   e Medical Professional
   f Labourer
   g Entrepreneur
   h Student
   i Skill Artisan

6 State/UT you reside in: _____
7 When you meet someone, you would prefer (in Check Boxes)

   i Shaking Hands
   ii. Hug
   iii First, Sanitise, then Shake Hands
   iv First, enquire about the person's Pandemic History
   v Greet verbally

8 Would you like to participate in (in Check Boxes)

    i   Get-together parties
    ii Hotels
    iii Pubs/Clubs
    iv Gyms
    v Hobby classes

9 Will you plan a trip after total unlock? (In Check Boxes)

    i   International trip within 6 months
    ii International trip within 1 year
    iii National trip within 6 months
    iv National trip within 1 year
    v Plan a trip immediately after air service resumes.

10 Are you worried about future uncertainty in life? Be it academic, familial, or professional life?

    Absolutely   Probably   Not Sure   Probably Not   Never

11 Are you anxious about getting optimum treatment for Coronavirus if it is found Positive?

    Absolutely   Probably   Not Sure   ProbablyNot   Never

12 Are you scared of getting Coronavirus?

    Absolutely   Probably   Not Sure   Probably Not   Never

13 Will you participate in religious events?

    Absolutely   Probably   Not Sure   Probably Not   Never

14 Will you continue cleaning and sanitising every item in your home?

    Absolutely   Probably   Not Sure   Probably Not   Never

15 Would you host your overseas relative or friend in your home?

    Absolutely   Probably   Not Sure   Probably Not   Never

16 Will you use public transport even in a rush?

    Absolutely   Probably   Not Sure   Probably Not   Never

17 Will you keep using masks as your routine dress-up?

    Absolutely   Probably   Not Sure   Probably Not   Never

18 Will you keep maintaining social distancing?

    Absolutely   Probably   Not Sure   Probably Not   Never

5 A Qualitative Enquiry of the Experience of Music Professionals during the COVID-19 Pandemic

Shalini Mittal, Tushar Singh, Durgesh Kumar Upadhyay, and Bhawna Tushir

India is a country of varying religions, dialects, traditions, customs, edibles, music, art, and architecture woven in a garland of patriotism and unity. One of the most distinguishing qualities of Indian culture is the Indian mindset, which can be characterised as welcoming, greeting, celebrating in a united way with immense affection and togetherness. Indian culture is quite rich not only because of its own heritage but also because it has assimilated the traits and cultures of the world (Chawla & Mohapatra, 2017). Modern historical and cultural research shows that Indian music has developed within a very complex interaction between people of different races and cultures. Indian music includes varieties of folk music, classical music, film music (Bollywood), Indian rock, and Indian pop. Every city in India has a genre of music associated with it. The Music of India has been evolving for ages with the changing realities of the society (Vedabala, 2016).

COVID-19 and the Indian Music Industry

The Indian music industry was formally established in the pre-independence era on 28 February 1936. After independence, North Indian classical music (Hindustani music) developed into varieties of new dimensions and angles. With the collapse of the British rule and the decline of the royal patronage, Indian classical musicians struggled for their basic survival needs along with the responsibility of keeping their family lineage alive. Moreover, musicians were exposed to the market forces and globalsation, which gave Indian music a different shape (Vedabala, 2016). Vedabala (2016) has listed the challenges before the Indian music industry in the 21st century. These are: (a) the numbers of musical performances, (b) its accountability in terms of the money the performer and program organisers earn; (c) popularity and fame of artists in India and abroad, (d) challenges in earning money by the music professionals in the national and international market, and (e) the challenges involved in making music available and acceptable to as many as possible. Before the COVID-19 pandemic, the Indian music industry was the second oldest and 20th largest music industry globally with its annual revenue of more than 155 million USD (Rehman, 2016).

However, the COVID-19 global pandemic resulted in disruptive, unusual, and uncertain conditions. Several studies have highlighted the impact of the COVID-19

DOI: 10.4324/9781003454984-6

pandemic on the emotional and psychological health of the general public as well as frontline health care professionals (Jaiswal et al., 2020), ranging from the psychological symptoms (i.e., feelings of anxiety, depression, insomnia, PTSD, suicide and suicidal ideations) (e.g., Xiong, et al., 2020; Tee et al., 2020; Que et al., 2020; Raj et al., 2021) to social reactions (i.e., stigma and discrimination (Bhanot et al., 2021), gender violence (Mittal & Singh, 2020; Maji et al., 2022) death and mourning (Das et al., 2021; Saraff et al., 2021).

The music industry also suffered due to the pandemic. As governments in various countries began imposing the lockdown to curtail the spread of the disease, several concerts, events, performances, and all other public gatherings were cancelled, creating severe disruptions in the entertainment industry. Botstein (2020) revealed that the audience for classical music in America had already been declining when the pandemic hit, making the future of the industry bleak in that country. The audience for classical music in America primarily comprises older people who are at the maximum risk of contracting COVID-19. Moreover, by the time the situation improved, many of these people became accustomed to and comfortable with the new technologies for listening to music. In fact, many researchers expected a rise in the consumption of online streaming services as the online social practice of live-streaming concerts has emerged as a popular outlet during the period of lockdown and social distancing (Vandenberg et al., 2020). However, Sim et al. (2020) observed a decline in digital streaming music consumption. Their research revealed that online music consumption declined by 12.5% on average, particularly in countries with a higher number of COVID-19 cases. Also, the recovery of such online music consumption was more remarkable in countries experiencing earlier alleviation of COVID-19.

Spiro et al. (2021) conducted a comprehensive study on performing arts professionals in the United Kingdom. They reported that music professionals experienced a decline in the workload due to the cancellation of work and events. They also expressed concern about the rapidly changing nature of work, the precariousness of freelancing, and the constraints of online working and working from home alongside the burden of domestic chores (Spiro et al., 2021). They also demonstrated that about 53% of participants reported a drop in their income and financial hardships (Spiro et al., 2021). Buldulku and Yesin (2020) have also highlighted that artists and performers generate far less revenue from online concerts than from live concerts.

Several other studies have highlighted the issues faced by music and art professionals during the current pandemic, such as techno-stress due to increased digital presence (De et al., 2020) and a decline in creativity during stressful circumstances (Duan et al., 2020) and have highlighted the importance of creativity and innovative practices in dealing with the problems posed by the pandemic (Cayari, 2020). Furthermore, studies have demonstrated that not only the stage performances but also teaching music has been affected badly during the pandemic. Ozer and Ustun (2020), for example, reported that the technical and connectivity issues adversely affect education, especially in applied courses such as music.

The Indian music industry was not spared from the effects of the COVID-19 pandemic. PHD Chamber of Commerce and Industry (PHDCCI) carried out research concerning the media and entertainment industry during the pandemic, reporting that recording studios are closing down in the music industry, creating a supply chain challenge. It was suspected that if the pandemic persists for a more extended period and keeps the population home-bound for more months, both music and TV companies in India would run out of new content to deliver to their audiences (2020). In fact, the Indian TV industry faced this challenge, and many TV channels either had to suspend their popular shows or had to telecast old episodes of previously popular TV programs.

Moreover, entertainment consumption in venues (encompassing sports, cinema, music, theatre, cultural fests, music events, *Jagrāta,* clubs, and many more) was significantly more impacted in the short term by COVID-19. Live music was another high-profile victim. Live streaming of concerts, online music training, and music-making in India are still at their nascent stage. Due to the COVID-19 pandemic, this sector in India had too little time to truly capitalise on the online music creation and dissemination opportunities.

Arguably, the music industry also suffered because of some additional issues. First, though music forms a significant part of our lives, it is not considered an essential part. The low to moderate level of essentiality of the music industry and the requirement of physical presence to experience it in concerts seriously impacted the stakeholders involved in this industry (Seetharaman, 2020). The fear of contraction of the disease was further intensified due to the expectation that brass and wind instruments would facilitate the propagation of infected airborne particles, which seems unlikely, according to the preliminary research by Moore and Cannaday (2020).

Though the COVID-19 had a differential impact on the different stakeholders in the music industry, depending on where they were in their careers and the nature of their work. As the music industry globally had undeniably suffered the brunt of the COVID-19 pandemic, it was extremely important to understand the impact of the COVID-19 pandemic on individual musicians, instrumentalists, and singers in India to provide practical solutions to overcome the sudden dip in the industry. Hence, the present research was conducted to explore qualitatively the experiences of Indian music professionals during the COVID-19 pandemic. More specifically, the present study aimed at investigating the following research questions:

- To understand the impact of the COVID-19 pandemic on music professionals in India.
- To understand the ways in which music professionals in India coped up with the challenges posed by the COVID-19 pandemic.

Method

Participants

For the present study, a call to invite volunteers for research participation was circulated among the music professionals via various social networks (e.g., WhatsApp groups, Facebook pages, and snowball sampling by initially identified participants). Efforts were made to identify participants who were at their early career stages. A total of 12 participants, including singers, instrumentalists, music teachers, composers, YouTube content creators residing in the State of Maharashtra, State of Uttar Pradesh, and the national capital of India, Delhi, were selected for the present study. Among the participants, seven were singers; three were instrumentalists, two were singer cum YouTube creators, and one participant was singer cum composer. Three participants were working as music teachers while others were freelancing in various capacities before the beginning of the pandemic. The age group of the participants ranged from 25 to 40 years. The average age of their professional experience was eight years. Table 5.1 shows the demographic details of the participants.

Procedure

Participants were contacted telephonically, and the purpose of this research was explained. To ensure the confidentiality of the participants, they were assigned codes (P1, P2, P3, ... , P12), and their names were not recorded in the data set. Rapport was established with the participants by holding a general conversation with them and explaining the current research's relevance. Semi-structured interviews were conducted from 15 July to 16 October 2020 to obtain the participants' experiences during the COVID-19 pandemic. Some of the questions asked included, "When did you first hear about the lockdown?", "How did you feel when you heard about the lockdown?", "In what ways has your professional life changed during the lockdown?" Although efforts were made to minimise the interference by the researcher, sometimes probes were used to elicit detailed responses. The participants were free to respond in Hindi or English. Later, all the narratives were

Table 5.1 The Demographic Details of the Participants

S. No.	Participant Code	Profession	Overall Professional Experience (years)	Month and Year of Interview
1.	P1	Singer/music teacher	15	October, 2020
2.	P2	Singer/music teacher	10	October, 2020
3.	P3	Singer/music teacher	5	October, 2020
4.	P4	Singer	5	September, 2020
5.	P5	Singer/composer/guitarist/ pianist	15	August, 2020
6.	P6	Singer	5	August, 2020
7.	P7	Singer/YouTube content creator	7	August, 2020
8.	P8	Singer/YouTube content creator	4	August, 2020
9.	P9	Sitar player	8	September, 2020
10.	P10	Singer	8	July, 2020
11.	P11	Singer	8	September, 2020
12.	P12	Tabla player	8	September, 2020

transcribed by the researcher. Later a bilingual expert unrelated to the research translated the Hindi narratives into English. The researcher reviewed the translations to ensure its appropriateness and consistency.

The study was conducted according to all the ethical guidelines as detailed in Helsinki's declarations and as mandated by APA in its ethical code of conduct for psychologists. In addition, all the participants provided recorded informed consent for their inclusion in this research and to record the conversations.

Analysis

The narratives were analysed using the six-step method of thematic content analysis proposed by Braun and Clarke (2006). In the first step of 'familiarising with the data, the narratives were read and re-read to gain familiarity. Initial notes highlighting the manifest content of the data were also made. The second step of 'generating initial codes' involved the meaningful organisation of the data. The initial codes were generated in this step, i.e., the data was broken down into smaller meaningful chunks. For instance, initial coding involved identifying initial codes, such as loss of jobs, no income from performances, and reduction in salaries. The third step involved 'searching themes.' There was some overlap in the second and third steps as by examining the initial codes, common patterns indicative of themes were identified. For instance, the mentioned initial codes were identified as a single theme of 'adverse financial impact.' In the fourth step, 'reviewing themes,' the preliminary themes identified were reviewed, modified, and developed. In step 5, 'defining themes', the essence of each theme was identified, refined, and emphasised on how each theme is relevant to the data. In the final step of 'writing-up, an attempt was made to write and explain the findings. For identifying the initial codes, the open coding method was used as the codes were not pre-determined. Instead, they were identified and developed during the process of analysis. The lead researcher carried out the analysis. Other researchers then reviewed the emergent themes, and once a consensus was reached, the common emergent themes were selected.

Results

Two major themes identified from the participants' narratives were 'impact on participating music professionals' and 'coping reactions.' The themes and subthemes that emerged in the narratives of the participants are set out in Table 5.2.

Impact on participating Music Professionals

Psychological Effects

Due to the COVID-19 pandemic, people were experiencing profound effects on mental health as it had several direct and indirect influences on an individual's mental health. Such impact on emotional and psychological health emerged in the form of feelings of anger and anxiety.

Table 5.2 The Common Themes Pertaining to the Experiences of Music Professionals during COVID-19 Pandemic and Imposition of Social Distancing Norms

S. No.	Themes	Subthemes	Indicators	Examples
1.	Impact on Music Professionals	Psychological Effects	Anxiety	"I was mostly anxious about contracting the disease. The condition in the hospitals seems to be bad. So, I feel worried." P6
			Anger	"I feel so irritated with this situation. Often that comes out on family members. But sometimes it happens. There is so much of uncertainty." P9
		Social Effects	Emotional Intimacy	"We are getting time with maa baba (mother and father) so they are also very happy." P4
			Estrangement	"We are used to going out all the time. Initially it was still fine. We thought lockdown would be temporary. But now we miss hanging out with friends. Phone cannot substitute that." P12
		Professional Effects	Work Load	"Teaching had now extended till 8 to 9 pm at night. We had to remain available on phone all the time." P3
			Adverse Financial Impact	"We cannot have stage shows so I have started teaching online. Because currently there is no earning from performances." P10
			Creativity Demands	"We had to think of something. What could we do despite sitting in our respective homes?" P4
			Helplessness	"Things have come to a standstill. But what can I do?" P10
			Audience Disconnect	"We feel that there is no platform to showcase our talents. Music students also feel that way." P1
			Digital Transformation Stress	"You keep getting instant feedback from the audience in a live stage performance. So, you can alter your performance accordingly." P5 "So many of us do not know how to use computers effectively. And we are forced to use it in the current situation. Youngsters still had been using it but for some of us holding classes and concerts online is very stressful."

(Continued)

Table 5.2 (Continued)

S. No.	Themes	Subthemes	Indicators	Examples
2	Coping Reactions	Coping Strategies used	Acceptance	"It is what it is. We must make the best of the current situation if we cannot change it." P12
				"We will have to change ourselves as per the situation. That's how it is in life." P1
			Habituation	"Initially it was difficult. I was not used to staying at home. But now I don't really feel the need to go out." P6
			Positive Life Orientation	"We are waiting. As soon as things get better, we are going to get back together for practice." P5
			Creative Thinking	"We our organizing online talent hunts for our music students. We will even launch a YouTube channel to showcase their talents. This is to ensure that they continue to get a platform." P1

Anxiety

Anxiety can be defined as negative feelings of apprehension. The conditions of uncertainty and the fear of contracting the disease inevitably led to feelings of anxiety among our participants. Several participants reported feeling anxious, for they felt that they might get infected with the coronavirus. For instance, one participant reported:

> "It does not feel safe to go out anymore. Constantly that thought of 'what if we get infected' keeps coming to the mind." P4

Anger

Anger refers to the feeling of annoyance and irritability. Though anger is a natural response to a frustrating situation, too much anger can have damaging effects on the person experiencing it. Participants reported feelings of anger towards the situation that were often displaced onto their family members. For example:

> "We are all confined together. Sometimes we get angry and irritated. Though we are not actually angry with them, it is vented out mostly on each other in the family." P4

Social Effects

The social distancing norms imposed during the COVID-19 pandemic have resulted in a paradoxical impact on the participants' social lives. Although, on the one hand, being able to spend more quality time at home with their immediate family members resulted in increased emotional intimacy, on the other hand, it also resulted in feelings of estrangement towards other people.

Emotional Intimacy

Emotional intimacy refers to improvement in emotional bonding and an increase in emotional closeness. People reported that before the pandemic, they could not spend quality time with their loved ones due to the daily hassles of life and hectic work schedules. However, at the time of the lockdown imposed during the COVID-19 pandemic, people were confined at homes. Consequently, they reported spending more time with their family members.

> "Earlier, because of my hectic schedule, I never used to get time with my family. But after a long time, I finally got sufficient time to spend with them. That's one positive outcome of this entire situation." P2

Estrangement

Estrangement can be defined as the loss of previously existing relations to the point of having negligible communication with others. Although the COVID-19 permitted people to spend more quality time with their immediate family members, for some of them, it resulted in cut-off from significant people in their lives, such as their friends, relatives, work peers, and colleagues.

> "I have literally become completely bored of staying at home. I am not getting to meet anyone; all the previous professional contacts have been lost." P9
> "I am feeling terrible as I could not go back to meet my parents in my hometown for the first time in years. Even they feel lonely." P1

Professional Effects

Though the increase in workload, financial loss, and digital transformation stress due to the COVID-19 pandemic have been experienced by several other professions, the nature of such influences seemed to be somewhat different for the participants of this study.

Increase in Work Load

During the current pandemic situation, participants experienced an increase in workload because in addition to the discontinuation of paid domestic help (common among the middle-income households in India to hire domestic help due to the availability of cheap labour) they had to acquaint themselves with new technology for performances. Some even began online teaching. More time was also spent coordinating with online event organisers and colleagues on the phone and other virtual platforms. Participants reported that:

> Work did increase because for safety purposes, we had to discontinue the domestic help. So, there was extra work. People were staying at home, so even the cooking process had become more elaborate. P2
> Earlier the classes would get over at 2 pm, and after that, we would be free to focus on our own practice and concerts. But now the class duration has increased. Some time is lost in ensuring whether you are audible to others and whether others are audible to you. Moreover, it is difficult to clear doubts online. Students keep calling up to clear that. Then making and uploading class videos is also time taking. P1
> Band practice has become so time-consuming. We are in our respective homes and trying to coordinate our vocals and instruments through video calling, but it is time-consuming and frustrating. Sometimes there is a lag; sometimes, there is a network issue. You put in so much time, and still, the outcome is not that great. I am eagerly waiting for this to get over so we can get back together and begin our practices. P5

Adverse Financial Impact

Participants in this research reported the severe impact of the pandemic on their earnings due to reduction in the sources of earning.

> Luckily, I am teaching at a school, so the financial impact is not that big. But still, since we are not having stage performances, so that has cut off our other sources of income. Earlier, we used to have a few stage performances or collaborations every now and then. That would lead to an added income. With that gone, we are managing our expenses accordingly. But others for whom the stage performances were the only way by which they could earn, it's real trouble. P2
>
> Artists have suffered major losses. There are some who have lost their primary source of income. Some are experiencing major cut-offs. Some have been reduced to a state where they are hoping that the government would provide some funding so that they can meet their ends meet. The COVID 19 has become the 'riches to rags' story for many wonderful artists. P1

Creativity Demands

COVID-19 has been increasingly placing demands on music professionals to be creative and innovative to maintain and revive their careers. Therefore, music professionals participating in this study had to quickly adapt and find alternatives to attract their audiences and maintain their professional visibility in addition to catering to their economic needs. Hence, several participants had adopted the ideas of online live concerts and YouTube channels. However, the availability of a variety of online content pressurised them to create unique content to maintain online visibility among their audiences. The following narrative indicated the creativity demands placed on the participants.

> Thing with an online forum is difficult. There is so much content out there that we have to be unique to attract the audience. You have to find something new in terms of either video, choice of songs, presentation, and such. You really have to put your mind to it and think out of the box. P5

Helplessness

Feelings of helplessness also emerged as a prominent theme among other influences of the COVID-19 pandemic. Helplessness can be defined as the feeling that one is unable to act effectively. These feelings were more prevalent among the music teachers who resorted to teaching through online platforms. For instance, participants said,

> As a teacher, I feel helpless that I am unable to teach my students all that I would want to. Due to lag and connectivity issues, I find it difficult to

interact online with my students. Some of them have started losing interest. Their career is at stake, and there is not much that I can do. P1

I feel irritated at times and sometimes sad that despite so much of hard work, I am unable to have the same kind of connect with the audience, the same kind of influence on them, and the same level of effectiveness with my students. And the problem is that I don't know what else can I do? P9

Audience Disconnect

The participants also expressed audience disconnect as a prominent theme among the various influences of COVID-19. The opportunity to perform on stage is extremely crucial for an artist's career as well as self-esteem (Parncutt & McPherson, 2002). However, the imposed lockdowns resulted in the cancellation of numerous events and concerts. Consequently, music professionals are experiencing a lack of platforms for showcasing their talents. This has become a cause of indirect psychological effects on them and was expressed among the participants in the form of low mood, anger, and irritation. This was indicated in the narratives of the participants, such as:

Biggest loss would be the loss of stage. I miss my performance days. When I cannot be on the stage, then I feel that my talent is being wasted. And I think that all artists might feel that way. The stage is what we live for. The absence of it kind of leaves a void. P11

Applause and appreciation from the audience are what the artist craves for. The sound of claps, that energy of a stage performance is missing. And it is like an addiction. You take that away, and it causes frustration. P4

In Facebook, people listen to the song and then scroll down. So yes, visibility is maintained, but we never know if this would be like this in a stage performance or whether the audience actually liked it. P7

There is a lag in an internet performance. So, they always react and clap 5 seconds later. That becomes distracting for our performance. Also, I include anecdotes in my performances. For a 5 minutes anecdote, I prepare 15 minutes of content. But you have to gauge the audience to know when to introduce which anecdote. So, though you can engross the audience through anecdotes online, you never get to know what they want at that moment. P5

Any day, I would prefer performing on stage to online concerts. Online I am not able to form that connects with the audience. P11

Digital Transformation Stress

Transitions of any kind can be stressful, including the transitions involving digitisation of work (Mikal et al., 2013). COVID-19 has accelerated the digital transformation of various professions and industries, including the music industry. The Music profession was primarily an experiential profession involving first-hand contact between the teacher-student, performer-audiences-collaborating artists.

However, the pandemic forced music professionals to digitalise their industry in a way that was never thought of. As a result, the speed and scale of digital transformation was reported to be stressful by many participants.

> The first one month was a total disaster. I hardly used to use a laptop. And mostly, it would be for watching a movie or writing something. And suddenly, I was forced to get acquainted with such complex software and applications for video calling. I will learn one thing, and the next day the icons used to get updated, and I will be lost again. It was stressful and even embarrassing in front of my students. P1
>
> I always thought that my table is the most important thing. But no. suddenly it's the laptop and the internet. I keep struggling with it. And I am still coping with it, and it's worst for my Guruji. I feel bad for him when he is forced to disrupt his classes for simple technical issues as he is unable to understand. P9

Coping Reactions

Coping Strategies Used

Sudden transitions and adjustments during the COVID-19 pandemic have been overwhelming for many people (Son et al., 2020), leading to significant personal and professional changes that have been stressful and influenced their physical and mental health (Fegert et al., 2020). Each individual attempts to cope with his/her situations and circumstances in his/her own way. Dominant coping reactions among music professionals that emerged after analysis of the narratives are discussed below.

Acceptance

Acceptance can be defined as the acknowledgement of the reality of the situation. It is a conscious choice wherein an individual acknowledges that the situation cannot be controlled, Thus, placing the individual in the best situation wherein they can focus on necessary changes. Several music professionals participating in the current research reported consciously acknowledging the reality of the present circumstances as a coping mechanism. For example, P5 says that

> Mumbai is so crowded that we have accepted that at least once we will get infected with Corona. As long as you have accepted that, you will be mentally prepared. It will not make you very anxious. And you will be on guard for the other problems that might come as a result of the pandemic. I believe this is how it is. P5

Habituation

Thompson and Spencer (1966) had described habituation in their landmark paper as a form of learning that reduces the magnitude of the stressful stimulus. In other

words, it refers to a decrease in response to stimulation following repeated exposure to it. During the initial phases of the COVID-19 pandemic and the imposed
lockdown, several individuals experienced intense anxiety, feelings of uncertainty,
anger, and even fear of contracting the disease. However, gradually these feelings declined as people got habituated to the prevailing conditions. The narratives
of several participants were indicative of habituation as a coping response. For
examples:

> The cases of COVID have not decreased, but the anxiety related to it surely
> has. We have become used to as far as this new way of life is concerned.
> So, it indeed is becoming the new normal. And also, I feel gradually I have
> reduced the amount of hand sanitizer that I am using. I make sure I don't
> touch things, but I am not as anxious as I was in the first couple of months. P3

Positive Life Orientation

Positive life orientation refers to an individual's strength to look forward and make
plans for the future. Positive life orientation has also been found to moderate the
relationship between perceived distress and coping (Pande & Tewari, 2016). Participants in the present study reported maintaining positive life orientations to deal
with stressful situation resulting due to the pandemic in narratives such as:

> I have decided to focus on the academic aspect of music until things become
> normal. This way, I will get time for my Ph.D. So, I practice alone, and then
> I utilize the rest of the time for working on my thesis. I believe that probably
> this is an opportunity for me to finish my academic work more quickly since
> there are no other distractions like concerts and social get-togethers. P6
>
> After lockdown gets over, I will start my music band. I have already con-
> tacted various artists who will be a part of it. I am getting to do all those
> things for which I usually do not have time. So, this is the bright side. Hope-
> fully, there will be some productive outcome if we try to utilize this time. P2

Creative Thinking

Several participants utilised creative thinking to find innovative solutions to revive
their careers and cope during the COVID-19 pandemic. This involved identifying
new platforms for performance and developing unique online content. For example,
music professionals have attempted to create videos and songs in collaboration with
each other from their respective homes. Yarbrough (1999) had discussed the possibility of a 'placeless society' where everything could be accessed via technology.
However, music professionals seemed to be turning this idea of a placeless society
into reality through creative thinking. For instance, one participant reported:

> We knew that even though everything has come to a standstill but still this time
> is important. So, we put our mind to it. We figured out how to record from our

respective homes and still make it feel like we are performing together. It was like a socially distanced virtual band. I collaborated with two other vocalists, one sitar player and a tabla (Tabor) player, recorded ourselves in our respective homes, and then later compiled it. It came out beautifully. P4

Discussion

The present study offers some significant findings pertaining to the impact of the COVID-19 pandemic on music professionals in India. Results of the study demonstrated that the music professionals in India experienced psychological symptoms, such as anxiety, anger, and feelings of helplessness over their career disruptions due to the COVID-19 pandemic. The mental health consequences of the pandemic have been studied widely across the globe which demonstrated that the pandemic had severely impacted the emotional and psychological health of the general public (e.g., Xiong et al., 2020; Tee et al., 2020; Que et al., 2020; Raj et al., 2021) as well as frontline health care professionals (Jaiswal et al., 2020). Several researches were indicative of the fact that the COVID-19 pandemic resulted in anxiety and fear about the post-pandemic career plans and outcomes (Parola, 2020; Mahmud et al., 2021). The feeling of helplessness was reported more by the professionals who possessed less than eight years of professional experience. They clearly mentioned the fact that professionally, they were still in their formative years and due to the COVID-19 restrictions, they were 'losing valuable time' which otherwise could have been used in their training and practice. It seemed that the stage at which the participants' career was (i.e., the extent to which they were professionally established) had played an essential role in contributing to the feelings of helplessness. Those with less professional experience seemed to experience more intense feelings of helplessness. These feelings of sadness and helplessness were also reported by music professionals who are working as music teachers and were teaching online. Participants reported that teaching music online was more complex and relatively ineffective when compared with conventional face-to-face music classes. They experienced several issues during online classes, including poor audio quality, lag in the audio, difficulty coordinating songs with all the students, connectivity issues, and many others. The music teachers found it difficult to point out the exact notes that were imperfect, and the students also found it challenging to sing with other students in a coordinated manner. This made the music learning process difficult and resulted in reduced interest in music classes. Consequently, they reported feeling low and helpless for not being able to contribute sufficiently to the students' learning and felt that the interest of the students also declined during online classes. According to Marshall et al. (2020), several teachers in their study reported witnessing barriers to student learning during online classes. According to Biasutti et al. (2021) music teachers reported teaching online to be a time-consuming endeavour. Ozer and Ustun (2020) also noted that the technical and connectivity issues experienced, adversely affected education, especially in applied courses such as music. The findings of this study, thus, not only confirmed such influences of the pandemic on Indian music professionals but also demonstrated that helplessness developed among the participants due to their inability to successfully contribute to their careers. This was a major concern among these music professionals which required immediate attention of the psychologists and mental health professionals. Moreover, Biasutti et al. (2021) further emphasised on the need for providing the music teachers with more institutional support to ensure their professional development.

The pandemic has had mixed consequences for the Indian music professionals' social experiences. While the participants experienced increased intimacy with their immediate family members, due to long lockdowns and social distancing measures they also experienced social disconnect from other important relations in their lives. Besides, the lockdown posed by the Indian government to siege the spread of coronavirus impacted the income and work-life balance of Indian music professionals. The income of professionals in the music and performing arts industry was aggregated below the national average, and artists used to work for lower wages due to the intrinsic value associated with the work (Cunningham, 2011; Taylor & Littleton, 2016). This was worsened by the pandemic and the resultant loss of employment as reported by the participants of the present study. Such an impact of COVID-19 on music professionals had been warned about in the very beginning of the pandemic (Sound Diplomacy, 2020). Increased subscribers to virtual music platforms, such as Apple Music indicated a rise in the consumption of music during the COVID-19 pandemic. Despite the increased consumption, the music professionals are struggling financially (Sound Diplomacy, 2020). Similar findings have been reported by Spiro et al. (2021), who demonstrated that about 53% of their participants reported a drop in their income and financial hardships. The Music industry is less telecommutable as it requires the physical presence of the performer and the audience to ensure the best possible experience for both the stakeholders. Not all music professionals could afford to produce soundtracks that can be sold online or in stores. With the cancellation of concerts around the globe, as reported by the music professionals participating in this research, they experienced a sudden dip in the revenue generated through such concerts. The cancellation of live performances resulted in the rise of popularity of novel formats, such as online concerts on social media platforms. However, the revenue generated through them remained meagre as the organisers paid them much less for online performances than for live performances. Though some participants began teaching in online music classes and workshops, the response to such efforts was not very enthusiastic due to the challenges associated with taking online classes. Thus, their income was considerably impacted during this pandemic. Furthermore, the need to record songs at home also created a demand for good quality equipment that can be very expensive and cannot be accessed by all music professionals. The differential impact of the pandemic was also observed among the music professionals participating in the study. Participants working as music teachers in the school reported feeling financially more secure during the COVID-19 as they continued to have at least one stable source of income.

In addition to the financial challenges, another professional challenge before the Indian music professionals was that of an increased workload that resulted in work-life imbalance which could be another reason for the mental health challenges faced by these professionals. The lockdown and containments measures imposed by the government forced the Indian musicians to take on increased responsibilities in the home and at the same time learn new skills related to carrying out professional activities in an online environment, which increased their overall workload. Thus, while other studies (e.g., Spiro et al., 2021) documented declines in traditional, established forms of professional music work, the experience of the participants of the current study indicated that paradoxically the reduction in traditional forms of professional work, coupled with increased domestic responsibility, actually lead to feelings of overwork, as the musicians also attempted to learn new skills very rapidly. These findings, however, must be compared cautiously because the present study qualitatively explored the pattern of work, both professional and personal, of the participating music professionals during the pandemic. In contrast, the other studies took into consideration primarily the professional work experience of the music professionals.

Several studies have highlighted the importance of being creative in times of adversity to deal with the adverse impacts of COVID-19 (e.g., Moss, 2020; Cayari, 2020). Research indicated a decline in creativity during stressful circumstances (Duan et al., 2020). An increase in stress, pressure to keep their careers alive, and a general reduction in creativity places high demands on the music profession-als to be creative. The continuous lockdowns required the music professionals to quickly adapt and find alternatives in order to ensure that their careers survive. Many of them resorted to the alternative of performing on virtual platforms, teach-ing, and conducting workshops online. This enabled the music professionals to resolve the issue of 'loss of stage.' However, this solution came with challenges of its own in the form of audience disconnect. The findings of research by Geeves et al. (2014) also indicated that professional musician's experience of their per-formance depended greatly on their connection with the audience, including the pre- and post-performance connection established with the audience. Findings of research by Kawase (2014) also revealed that the audience's facial expressions, gaze, and verbal expressions were perceived as important by the performers and the audience. The music industry, like any other source of entertainment, offers the best experience through physical presence. However, the artists found it chal-lenging to engage the audiences in the same way because they were able to do so during live performances. Participants reported that they could alter and 'lift' their performance up based on the immediate feedback received from the audience in the form of non-verbal cues. These cues were not available in online performances. Moreover, online performances came with challenges of their own, resulting from connectivity issues and lag in audio-visuals that can be very distracting for the art-ist. Also, research indicated that though music is reproducible in soft copy and is cheaply available on several online software, it created a disconnect between the music as a product and music professional as its creator (Sound Diplomacy, 2020).

Schwarz et al. (2020) acknowledged that though COVID-19 pandemic resulted in adaptation of digital formats even in academics and research, it fails to substitute physical interaction completely. They further pointed out an increase in the levels of stress resulting from such digital transformations due to blurring of personal and professional space. Vial (2019) too had emphasised that digital transformation as a process can cause disruptions. De et al. (2020) have also highlighted the possible experience of techno-stress due to increased digital presence. The stress was worsened due to the lack of skill and culture for digitisation among the music professionals. The current pandemic accelerated the digital transformation process to keep the businesses and careers afloat by the participants of the present research. However, there were several associated challenges, such as the issue of transferring a course online, effectiveness of the course, skills of the online teacher (Fawns et al., 2020), and the issue of generating the same amount of revenue from online concerts as from the live concerts (Buldulku & Yesin, 2020). These challenges associated with the sudden transitions are stressful, as pointed out by the current research participants. The participants reported increased use of social networking sites for uploading videos and maintaining their visibility as an artist. In addition to that, video conferencing applications, such as 'Zoom', 'Google Meet' and 'Microsoft Teams' have also been forced upon them. Various participants reported this transition to be stressful.

The psychological, social, and professional challenges faced by the Indian music professional created several unending and ambiguous challenges before them. An efficient and effective adoption to these challenges was necessary for them to survive under these extreme circumstances. The music professionals, thus, utilised several coping resources to deal with these challenges. These were active acceptance, habituation, positive life orientation, and creative thinking. Active acceptance has been found to be an adaptive strategy that results in positive psychological outcomes (Nakamura & Orth, 2005). According to Kishita and Shimada (2011), acceptance helps in reducing subjective stress and improves task performance. According to Polizzi et al. (2020), acceptance-based coping in the face of the pandemic allows one to accept that the fear of the virus exists. Acceptance of this fear within the realistic limits provides for an adaptive response. They further reported that acceptance may also help increase distress tolerance and encourage taking goal directed actions to cope with COVID-19 pandemic. Bishop et al. (2006) reported that an inherent part of mindfulness is acceptance that can help in accepting the transient nature of the ever-changing life circumstances when dealing with grief and loss (Olendzki, 2013).

According to Saha et al. (2020), habituation reduced symptomatic psychosocial expression during COVID-19 over time. Other studies, too, have highlighted the effectiveness of habituation in lowering PTSD symptoms (Bodour et al., 2017), anxiety, and fear (Maples-Keller & Rauch, 2020) and thus supported the findings of the present study. According to Xiong et al. (2021) habituation to stressful situations played a protective role against the negative influences of the COVID-19 pandemic among Chinese medical students. Although, some researches were indicative of the detrimental impact of COVID-19 on the career planning of individuals due to the experience of acute stress (Zhang et al., 2021), participants of the present study reported that they are utilising these times to plan for the future and work on plans that were delayed due to the scarcity of time. The role of creativity in coping is well established. According to Metzl (2009), creative thinking increases resilience and predict coping abilities by reducing the problematic stress response. Furthermore, as Kapoor and Kaufman (2020) rightly noted, creativity can help find meaning during these times of crisis. Larner and Blow (2011) have reported that individuals with post-traumatic stress disorder utilise meaning focused coping. Both Frankl's (1946) and Lifton's (1979, 2011) conceptions have indicated towards the role of creativity in finding meaning. Participants of the present study also used creativity to cope with the constraints due to COVID-19.

Though everyone was unprepared for dealing with the sudden onset of a pandemic, the brunt of it was worse for certain professions that were not telecommutable in nature. This was also the case for the music professionals as experiencing of the music and forming a connection with the audience is crucial to their work. Nonetheless, based on the findings of the present study it is suggested to build a resilience plan for the music professionals to protect them from the negative influences of the COVID-19 pandemic. One of the primary measures that can be adopted is to ensure an enhanced availability of funding for the music professionals. The *Kala Sanskriti Vikas Yojana Scheme* of the Ministry of Culture, India, had schemes to provide financial assistance to the artists in the field of performing arts (Ministry of Culture, 2019–2020). However, this financial assistance was not sufficient to safeguard the interests of the music professionals. Sound Diplomacy (2020) pointed out the importance of music for the economic, social and even mental health of people. In fact, there is extensive research to suggest that music can also reduce the crime rate in a community (Daykin et al., 2013; Rentfrow, 2012). Considering these positive influences of music, efforts are needed to prioritise the field of music in policy frameworks. Also, government often subjects the music professionals to genre discrimination and provides financial assistance mostly to music professionals that are engaged in traditional forms of music. To ensure that all music professionals are buffered against the harmful influences of the pandemic and the possible future crisis situations, government must try to encourage diverse genres of music.

Conclusion

COVID-19 had led to adverse effects on various aspects of life globally. The music industry, too, had experienced its dramatic and damaging consequences in the form of creativity demands, increase in workload, financial loss, audience disconnect, and many others, which contributed to direct and indirect mental health issues. These impacts, however, were not the same but are different for different music professionals due to several reasons. For instance, the nature of digital transformation stress was different for those performing in online concerts than those teaching music in online classes. Also, the adverse financial impact was worse for some participants. At the same time, those who were also music teachers and stage performers experienced some financial stability as they had at least one continuous source of income. The amount of work experience held by the music professionals also seemed to had an influence over their experience during the COVID-19 pandemic and the period of imposed lockdown. While those who were already well established in their careers got opportunities for online concerts, other participants thought they were losing valuable time.

The present research findings are significant as they contribute to our understanding of the differential impact of COVID-19 on music professionals participating in the study. The music industry is vast, with several people gaining employment from it. However, the pandemic has adversely affected the industry along with those who are a part of it. By describing the nature of such an impact, the current study's findings can help effectively plan the future of the industry and find solutions. The study also provides an insight into the pros and cons of the mitigating actions taken by the music professionals participating in the current research during the pandemic. Based on the findings the present research has also suggested to develop a resilience plan to protect the music professionals in the current and future crisis situations. Despite giving an insight into the experiences of the music professionals during the COVID-19 pandemic, the results of this research have some limitations, and hence they must be interpreted with caution. Being a qualitative study, these findings present a great insight into the experiences of the study participants. However, since every individual responds differently to stressful situations, the current research findings apply only to the music professionals participating in this research. Therefore, studies replicating the current research are required to further validate the present research findings and allow for further generalisation. It is also interesting to note that none of the participants of the present research expressed concern about the long-lasting impact of COVID-19 on the respiratory system, as pointed out in some studies (Vance et al., 2021).

References

Biasutti, M., Antonini Philippe, R., & Schiavio, A. (2021). Assessing teachers' perspectives on giving music lessons remotely during the COVID-19 lockdown period. *Musicae Scientiae, 26*(3). https://doi.org/10.1177/1029864921996033

Bishop, R. S., Lau, M., Shaphiro, S., Carlson, L., Anderson, N. D., Carmody, J., et al. (2006). Mindfulness: A proposed operational definition. *Clinical Psychology: Science and Practice, 11*, 230–241.

Bhanot, D, Singh, T, Verma, S. K., & Sharad, S. (2021). Stigma and discrimination during COVID-19 pandemic. *Frontiers in Public Health, 8*, 577018. https://doi.org/10.3389/fpubh.2020.577018

Badour, C. L., Flanagan, J. C., Gros, D. F., Killeen, T., Pericot-Valverde, I., Korte, K. J., Allan, N. P., & Back, S. E. (2017). Habituation of distress and craving during treatment as predictors of change in PTSD symptoms and substance use severity. *Journal of Consulting and Clinical Psychology, 85*(3), 274–281. https://doi.org/10.1037/ccp0000180

Botstein, L. (2020). The future of music in America: The challenge of COVID-19 pandemic. *The Musical Quarterly, 102*(4), 351–360.

Braun, V., & Clarke, V. (2006). Using thematic analysis in psychology. *Qualitative Research in Psychology, 3*, 77–101.

Buldulku, Y., & Yesin, M. M. (2020). Media, sports and the entertainment industry in the post pandemic period. In M. Seker, A. Ozer, & C. Korkut (Eds.), *Reflections on the pandemic in the future of the world* (pp. 961–986). Ankara: Turkish Academy of Sciences.

Cayari, C. (2020). Popular practices for online musicking and performance: Developing creative dispositions for music education and the internet. *Journal of Popular Music Education, 5*(3), 295–312.

Chawla, H., & Mohapatra, H. (2017). Indian culture and globalization. *International Inventive Multidisciplinary Journal, 5*(3), 9–16.

Cunningham, S., 2011. Developments in measuring the "creative" workforce. *Cultural Trends, 20*, 25–40.

Das, S., Singh, T., Varma, R., & Arya, Y. K. (2021). Death and mourning process in frontline health care professionals and their families during COVID-19. *Frontiers in Psychiatry, 12*, 624428. https://doi.org/10.3389/fpsyt.2021.624428

Daykin, N., De Viggiani, N., Pilkington, P., & Yvonne, M. (2013). Music making for health, well-being and behaviour change in youth justice settings: A systematic review. *Health Promotion International, 28*(2), 197–210.

De, R., Pandey, N. & Pal, A. (2020). Impact of digital surge during Covid-19 pandemic: A viewpoint on research and practice. *International Journal of Information Management, 55*, 102171. https://doi.org/10.1016/j.ijinfomgt.2020.102171.

Duan, H., Wang, X., Hu, W., & Kounios, J. (2020). Effects of acute stress on divergent and convergent problem-solving. *Thinking & Reasoning, 26*, 68–86.

Fawns, T., Jones, D., & Aitkin, G. (2020). Challenging assumptions about 'moving online' in response to COVID 19 and some practical advice. *MedEd Publish*, 1–18. https://doi.org/10.15694/mep.2020.000083.1

Fegert, J. M., Vitiello, B., Plener, P. L., & Clemens, V. (2020). Challenges and burden of the Coronavirus 2019 (COVID-19) pandemic for child and adolescent mental health: A narrative review to highlight clinical and research needs in the acute phase and the long return to normality. *Child and Adolescent Psychiatry and Mental Health, 14*, 20.

Frankl, V. E. (1946). *Man's search for meaning.* Boston, MA: Beacon Press.

Geeves, A. M., McIlwain, D. J., & Sutton, J. (2014). Seeing yellow: 'Connection' and routine in professional musicians' experience of music performance. *Psychology of Music, 44*(2), 183–201. https://doi.org/10.1177/0305735614560841.

Jaiswal, A., Singh, T., & Arya, Y. K. (2020). "Psychological antibodies" to safeguard frontline healthcare warriors mental health against COVID-19 pandemic-related psychopathology. *Frontiers in Psychiatry, 11*, 590160. https://doi.org/10.3389/fpsyt.2020.590160

Kapoor, H., & Kaufman, J. C. (2020). Meaning-making through creativity during COVID 19. *Frontiers in Psychology, 11*.

Kawase, S. (2014). Importance of communication cues in music performance according to performers and audience. *International Journal of Psychological Studies, 6*(2), 49–64.

Kishita, N., & Shimada, H. (2011). Effects of acceptance-based coping on task performance and subjective stress. *Journal of Behaviour Therapy and Experimental Psychiatry, 42*(1), 6–12.

Larner, B., & Blow, A. (2011). A model of meaning-making coping and growth in combat veterans. *Review of General Psychology, 15*(3), 187–197.

Lifton, R. J. (2011). *Witness to an extreme century: A memoir.* Mumbai: Free Press.

Lifton, R. J. (1979). *The broken connection.* New York: Simon & Schuster.

Maji, S., Bansod, S., & Singh, T. (2022). Domestic violence during COVID-19 pandemic: The case for Indian women. *Journal of Community & Applied Social Psychology, 32*(3), 374–381.

Mahmud, M. S., Talukder, M. U., & Rahman, S. M. (2021). Does 'Fear of COVID-19' trigger future career anxiety? An empirical investigation considering depression from COVID-19 as a mediator. *The International Journal of Social Psychiatry, 67*(1), 35–45.

Maples-Keller, J. L., & Rauch, S. A. M. (2020). Habituation. In J. S. Abramowitz & S. M. Blakey (Eds.), *Clinical handbook of fear and anxiety: Maintenance processes and treatment mechanisms* (pp. 249–263). American Psychological Association. https://doi.org/10.1037/0000150-014

Marshall, D. T., Shannon, D. M., & Savanna, L. M. (2020). How teachers experienced the COVID-19 transition to remote instruction. *Phi Delta Kappan, 102*(3), 46–50.

Metzl, E. S. (2009). The role of creative thinking in resilience after hurricane Katrina. *Psychology of Aesthetics, Creativity, and the Arts, 3*(2), 112–123.

Mikal, J. P., Rice, R. E., Abeyta, A., & DeVilbiss, J. (2013). Transition, stress and computer-mediated social support. *Computers in Human Behaviour, 29*(5), A40–A53. https://doi.org/10.1016/j.chb.2012.12.012.

Ministry of Culture. (2019–2020). *Annual report*. Retrieved July 22, 2021, from https://www.indiaculture.nic.in/annual-reports

Mittal, S., & Singh, T. (2020). Gender-based violence during COVID-19 pandemic: A mini-review. *Frontiers in Global Women's Health, 1*, 4. https://doi.org/10.3389/fgwh.2020.00004

Moore, T. R., & Cannaday, A. E. (2020). Do "brassy" sounding musical instruments need increased safe distancing requirements to minimize the spread of COVID-19? *Journal of Acoustical Society of America, 148*, 2096.

Nakamura, Y. M., & Orth, U. (2005). Acceptance as a coping reaction: Adaptive or not? *Swiss Journal of Psychology, 64*(4), 281–292.

Olendzki, A. (2013). The roots of mindfulness. In: C. K. Germer & P. R. Gulton (Eds.), *Mindfulness and psychotherapy* (2nd ed.) (pp. 242–261). New York: Guildford Press.

Ozer, B., & Ustun, E. (2020). Evaluation of students' views on the COVID-19 distance education process in music departments of fine arts faculties. *Asian Journal of Education and Training, 6*, 556–558.

Pande, N., & Tewari, S. (2016). Understanding coping with distress due to physical disability. *Psychology and Developing Societies, 23*(2), 177–209.

Parncutt, R., & McPherson, G. (Eds.). (2002). *The science and psychology of music performance: Creative strategies for teaching and learning.* Oxford: Oxford University Press.

Parola, A. (2020). Novel coronavirus outbreak and career development: A narrative approach into the meaning for Italian university graduates. *Frontiers in Psychology, 11*. https://doi.org/10.3389/fpsyg.2020.02255

Polizzi, C., Lynn, S. J., & Perry, A. (2020). Stress and coping in the time of COVID 19: Pathways to resilience and recovery. *Clinical Neuropsychiatry, 17*(2), 59–62.

Que, J., Shi, L., Deng, J., Liu, J., Zhang, L., Wu, S., et al. (2020). Psychological impact of the COVID-19 pandemic on healthcare workers: A cross-sectional study in China. *General Psychiatry, 33*(3).

Raj, S., Ghosh, D., Singh, T., Verma, S. K., & Arya, Y. K. (2021). Theoretical mapping of suicidal risk factors during the COVID-19 pandemic: A mini-review. Frontiers in Psychiatry, *11*, 589614. https://doi.org/10.3389/fpsyt.2020.589614

Rehman, S. (2016). The role of music in Hindi cinema. *Synergy, 12*(2), 314–329.

Rentfrow, P. J. (2012). The role of music in everyday life: Current directions in the social psychology of music. *Social and Personality Psychology Compass, 6*(5), 402–416.

Saha, K., Torous, J., Caine, E. D., & Choudhury, M. (2020). Psychosocial effects of the COVID 19 pandemic: Large scale quasi experimental study on social media. *Journal of Medical Internet Research, 22*(11), e22600.

Saraff, S., Singh, T., & Biswal, R. (2021). Coronavirus disease 2019: Exploring media portrayals of public sentiment on funerals using linguistic dimensions. *Frontiers in Psychology, 12*, 626638. https://doi.org/10.3389/fpsyg.2021.626638

Schwarz, M., Scherrer, A., Hohmann, C., Heiberg, J., Brugge, A., & Nunez-Jimenez, A. (2020). COVID 19 and the academy: It is time for going digital. *Energy Research and Social Science, 68*, 101684.

Seetharaman, P. (2020). Business model shifts: Impact of COVID-19. *International Journal of Information Management, 54*, 102173.

Sim, J., Cho, D., Hwang, Y., & Telang, R. (2020). Virus shook the streaming star: Estimating the COVID-19 impact on music consumption. *Marketing Science*. SSRN: https://papers.ssrn.com/sol3/papers.cfm?abstract_id=3649085

Son, C., Hegde, S., Smith, A., Wang, X., & Sasangohar, F. (2020). Effects of COVID-19 on college students' mental health in the United States: Interview survey study. *Journal of Medical Internet Research, 22*(9), e21279. https://doi.org/10.2196/21279

Sound Diplomacy. (2020). *Music cities – resilience handbook*. Retrieved July 22, 2021, from https://www.sounddiplomacy.com/better-music-cities

Spiro, N., Perkins, R., Kaye, S., Tymosuzk, U., Mason-Bertrand, A., Cossette, I., et al. (2021). The effects of COVID-19 lockdown 1.0 on working patterns, income, and wellbeing among performing arts professionals in the United Kingdom. *Frontiers in Psychology, 11*, 1–17.

Taylor, S., & Littleton, K. (2016). *Contemporary identities of creativity and creative work.* New York: Routledge.

Tee, M. L., Tee, C. A., Anlacan, J. P., Aligam, K., Reyes, P., Kuruchittham, V., & Ho, R. C. (2020). Psychological impact of COVID-19 pandemic in the Philippines. *Journal of Affective Disorders, 277*, 379–391.

Thompson, R. F., & Spencer, W. A. (1966). Habituation: A model phenomenon for the study of neuronal substrates of behavior. *Psychological Review, 73*(1), 16–43.

Vance, D., Shah, P., & Sataloff, R. T. (2021). COVID 19: Impact on the musician and returning to singing: A literature review. *Journal of Voice, 37*(2), 292.e1–292.e8.

Vandenberg, F., Berghman, M., & Schaap, J. (2020). The 'lonely raver': Music livestreams during COVID-19 as a hotline to collective consciousness? *European Societies, 23*, 5141–5152.

Vedabala, S. (2016). Indian classical music in a globalized world. *Sangeet Galaxy, 5*(1), 3–9.

Vial, G. (2019). Understanding digital transformation: A review and a research agenda. *The Journal of Strategic Information Systems, 28*. https://doi.org/10.1016/j.jsis.2019.01.003.

Xiong, J., Lipsitz, O., Nasri, F., Lui, L. M. W., Gill, H., Phan, L., et al. (2020). Impact of COVID-19 pandemic on mental health in the general population: A systematic review. *Journal of Affect Disorders, 277*, 55–64.

Xiong, P., Ming, W., Zhang, C., Bai, J., Luo, C., Cao, W., et al. (2021). Factors influencing mental health among Chinese medical and non-medical students in the early stage of the COVID 19 pandemic. *Frontiers in Public Health, 9*, 603331.

Yarbrough, C. (1999). What should be the relationship between schools and other sources of music learning? In Vision 2020: The Housewright Symposium on the Future of Music Education. National Association for Music Education. https://nafme.org/wp-content/files/2015/12/16-WhatShouldBetheRelationship-between-Schools-and-Other-Sources-of-Music-Learning.pdf

Zhang, L., Qi, H., Wang, L., Wang, F., Huang, J., Li, F., & Zhang, Z. (2021). Effects of COVID 19 pandemic on acute stress disorder and career planning among healthcare students. *International Journal of Mental Health Nursing, 30*(4), 907–916.

6 Spiritual Dispositional Coping and Health Hardiness on Stress and Related Illnesses

Aftermath COVID-19

Ishanpreet Kaur Toor and Kritika Rastogi

Introduction

The pandemic has stressed the international system and tested established institutions beyond their limits. It led to a huge impact on various facets of our lives, including financial, educational, socio-economic, and psychological (Grover et al., 2020; Ibn-Mohammed et al., 2021; Joshi et al., 2020; Sharma et al., 2021). Determinants like social isolation, worry about contracting the coronavirus, financial setbacks, and fears about health and safety all contributed to the heightening of negative emotional responses (Fofana et al., 2020; Heffner et al., 2021; Porcelli, 2020). These emotions, in turn, led to adverse effects, resulting in psychological conditions like depression, anxiety, and stress (Elbay et al., 2020). Post-pandemic stress disorder (PPSD), a mental health condition, emerged as a result of the excruciating amount of stress experienced during the pandemic. Owen O'Kane in 2021 introduced this condition, which is said to be very similar to post-traumatic stress disorder (PTSD). The symptoms of PPSD include intrusive thoughts, avoidance behaviours, hyperarousal, and negative changes in mood and thoughts (Grajek et al., 2022; Łaskawiec et al., 2022). This indicates the profundity of people's stress during a pandemic, making them more susceptible to chronic stress-related diseases (Tsamakis et al., 2020). Another health complexity that has arisen is "Long COVID" (post-acute sequelae of SARS-CoV-2 infection, or PASC), which refers to symptoms that continue for several weeks or months after the acute phase of a coronavirus infection (Munblit et al., 2022; Parotto et al., 2023). This pertains to mental, cognitive, and physical health and multisystem complications that include the immune, musculoskeletal, nervous, cardiovascular, renal, gastrointestinal, and respiratory systems. As a result, taking care of one's psychological well-being and health has become an absolute necessity.

Research suggests a potent relationship between health and spirituality (Koenig, 2004; Sloan et al., 1999). So much evidence exists that it incorporates the spiritual dimension in the biopsychosocial framework (Hatala, 2012; Sulmasy, 2002). The new medical framework of biopsychosocial-spiritual indicates that all these facets are essential to overall recovery and coping with a disease. Balboni and colleagues (2022), who conducted a study at Harvard University led by a Delphi panel of multidisciplinary experts, concluded that spirituality is crucial for the future of

DOI: 10.4324/9781003454984-7

whole-person-centred care in the healthcare industry. It was pointed out that participation in spiritual community services has been associated with healthier lifestyles, including greater longevity, a reduced likelihood of depression and suicide, and lower rates of substance abuse (Balboni et al., 2022).

People used numerous spiritual and religious coping strategies to deal with the challenges during the pandemic. In India and Nigeria, positive religious coping was seen during the pandemic in cross-national survey research (Fatima et al., 2022). Individuals have adopted various coping methods during the pandemic and begun engaging in practices, such as mindfulness, yoga, herb consumption, and meditation (Behan, 2020; Khanna et al., 2021; Zope et al., 2021). The understanding is that engaging in behaviours that prevent us from catching diseases and maintaining health plays a vital role in subduing the effects of the pandemic.

Another important way to deal with the pandemic's consequences is through hardiness. Hardiness is a concept that evolved in 1979 from the work of psychologist Suzanne C. Kobasa, stating three characteristics: commitment, control, and challenge. As a result, health hardiness is analogous to these components when applied to health. Bartone et al. (2022) conducted research in Canada to understand the effects of COVID-19 on mental health. The study confirmed that the pandemic significantly increased anxiety and depression symptoms, also suggesting that individuals with high hardiness have decreased stress and anxiety, thus concluding that hardiness is a protective factor.

The chapter dives deep into the potential protective factors against the negative impact of stress on psychological and physical health. It also sheds light on the effects of aggravated stress on our physical health and the underlying stress-related diseases. It aims to elucidate the pandemic's effects, reinforce the connection between spirituality and health hardiness, and discuss how strengthening one's health hardiness and instilling spiritual traits will help one cope with the public health crisis effectively.

Understanding Stress-Related Illnesses in the Aftermath of COVID-19

Negative Emotional Response

Emotions are intricate psychological states involving a range of physiological and cognitive responses to a specific stimulus or situation. Physical sensations, such as alterations in heart rate, breathing, and muscle tension, frequently accompany emotions. Emotions can be ascribed to positive and negative emotions, such as joy, sorrow, rage, fear, and love. Emotions can influence our thoughts, behaviours, and decision-making processes (Marcus, 2003; Niedenthal & Ric, 2017).

The ramifications of this long-duration pandemic caused fear, uncertainty, and isolation. All this affected people's emotional and psychological well-being, further impacting their physical health. Various measures adopted by the government administration, such as social distancing, lockdowns, and travel restrictions, led to isolation, negatively affecting health and well-being. The widespread feeling of

Table 6.1 According to a Systematic Review and Meta-Analysis by Salari et al. (2020)

Psychological Disorders	Continent	Number of Articles	Sample Size	I^2	Egger's Test	Prevalence (95% CI)
Anxiety	Asia	13	54,596	99.2	0.136	32.9 (28.2–37.9)
	Europe	3	8,341	98.8	0.272	23.8 (27.3–44.1)
Depression	Asia	10	35,688	99.5	0.224	35.3 (27.3–44.1)
	Europe	3	8,341	99.2	0.104	32.4 (21.6–45.5)
Stress	Asia	3	2,758	96.3	0.229	27.9 (19.7–37.8)
	Europe	2	6,316	98.5	–	31.9 (23.1–42.2)

loneliness contributed to anxiety, depression, stress, and other health conditions (Fofana et al., 2020; Palgi et al., 2020)

According to Table 6.1, during the pandemic, the prevalence of stress was 31.9%, anxiety was 32.9%, and depression was 35.3% in Asia. Whereas in Europe, the prevalence of stress was 27.9%, depression was 32.4%, and anxiety was 23.8%, which is comparably lower than in Asia. The research suggested that appropriate psychological strategies, techniques, and interventions can be developed to maintain and improve the general population's mental health during the COVID-19 pandemic (Salari et al., 2020).

These negative emotions are further responsible for escalating stress during this period. Stress is a response that occurs when someone faces a threatening or challenging situation. It is an evolutionary mechanism wherein the body faces or flees from the stressor. Due to this extended period of sadness, despair, and loneliness, individuals' bodies can enter a state of chronic stress. Chronic stress is a condition that occurs due to prolonged stress that has persisted over an extended period (Wheaton, 1997). Chronic stress is detrimental to both psychological and physical health. It can become an onset for developing and contracting various diseases and illnesses.

Stress-Related Illness

It is essential to understand what stress is and its physiological effects. The experience of stress elicits a complex physiological response involving the nervous and endocrine systems (Charmandari et al., 2005). The stress response in the body involves two distinct systems – the first is the SAM axis, i.e., the sympathetic adrenomedullary, which is responsible for stimulating the sympathetic nervous system (fight or flight), producing noradrenaline and adrenaline. Simultaneously, the endocrine system that activates during the stress response is the HPA axis, known as the hypothalamus-pituitary adrenocortical, which leads to the secretion of a chemical known as cortisol (stress hormone) (Chu et al., 2022). The optimal amount of cortisol is essential for the body as it helps defend itself during an adverse situation (Godoy et al., 2018).

Further health and disease implications are associated with the dysregulation of stress reactivity. There has been a connection between the

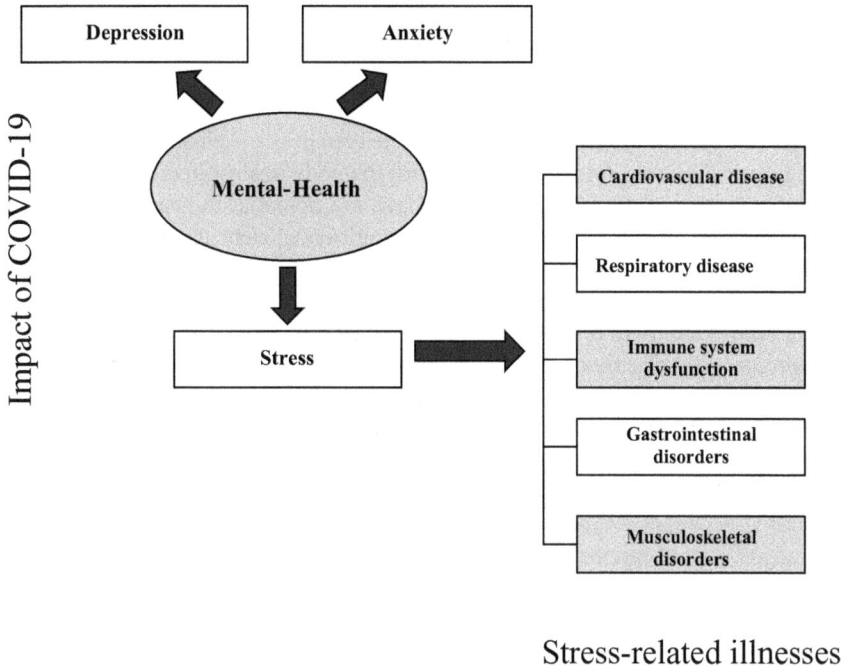

Stress-related illnesses

Figure 6.1 Showing the Relationship between the Impact of COVID-19 and Stress-Related Illnesses.

excessive reactivity of the sympathetic-adrenal-medullary (SAM) system and the hypothalamic-pituitary-adrenal (HPA) axis to psychological stresses and the development of cardiovascular disease, metabolic disorders, and immunological dysfunction (Glaser & Kiecolt-Glaser, 2005; Lee et al., 2015; Steptoe & Kivimäki, 2012). These systems' blunted reactivity has been linked to the emergence of depression, anxiety, and chronic pain (Turner et al., 2020).

Figure 6.1 shows that the pandemic brought about mental health problems, such as anxiety, depression, and stress. Prolonged exposure to stress causes stress-related illnesses, including cardiovascular disease, respiratory disease, immune dysfunction, gastrointestinal disorders, and musculoskeletal disorders (Liu et al., 2017; Salleh, 2008).

The following are major stress-related diseases:

1 *Cardiovascular diseases (CVD)* refer to conditions affecting the cardiac system or blood vessels. It is caused by fatty deposits inside the arteries, known as atherosclerosis, which also increases the risk of blood clots. Studies suggest that high cortisol levels from long-term stress can increase blood cholesterol, triglycerides, blood sugar, and blood pressure (Kelsall et al., 2020).
2 *Respiratory conditions:* These affect the functioning of the lungs and other associated organs. These conditions include asthma, chronic obstructive pulmonary

disease (COPD), pneumonia, and lung cancer. Stress stimulates adrenal glands to release cortisol and adrenaline, increasing respiration rate and making breathing more difficult for those with the above underlying conditions (Aich et al., 2009).

3 *Immune system dysfunction:* The immune system is a sophisticated network of organs, cells, and proteins that safeguard the body against invading pathogens. Dysfunctions of the immune system have the potential to result in the manifestation of allergic conditions, immunological deficiencies, and autoimmune pathologies. Prolonged exposure to stress can result in immune system dysregulation, thereby triggering the reactivation of latent viruses and compromising the body's ability to regulate viral activity (Morey et al., 2015).

4 *Autoimmune diseases* are medical conditions where the immune system accidentally harms the body's healthy cells, tissues, or organs. Systemic Lupus erythematosus Rheumatoid arthritis, Hashimoto, Crohn's disease, and a few thyroid diseases are examples of these types. In a study, researchers evaluated the likelihood of developing an autoimmune illness in individuals diagnosed with stress-related conditions. According to the study, people diagnosed with a stress-related problem are more at risk of developing multiple autoimmune disorders (Song et al., 2018).

5 *Gastrointestinal problem:* Stress can disturb the body's digestive system, leading to stomach ulcers, acid reflux, irritable bowel syndrome, and irritable bowel disorder. The cardiovascular system intensifies during stressful times, diverting blood from the gastrointestinal tract. People under stress frequently have issues like constipation, nausea, and irritable bowel syndrome because their gastrointestinal tract does not receive adequate blood flow (Mönnikes et al., 2001).

6 *Musculoskeletal disorders* constitute multiple conditions impacting bones, joints, muscles, and connective tissues. The musculoskeletal system is in a more permanent state of constriction with chronic stress. Over time, persistent muscle tension can result in injury and chronic pain, including back and neck pain, and may even cause secondary disorders, such as migraines (Hämmig, 2020).

Spiritual Dispositional Coping

Spirituality

The word "spirituality" originates from the Latin *spiritus,* which means "breath, courage, soul, life, and includes the ethereal idea of the spirit. It is the English equivalent of the Greek word *pneuma,* connected to words like inspire, expire, and breathe" (Buck, 2006). "Spirituality" is frequently called meaning, worth, transcendence, connection, and human development. The Western ideas about having faith in God and feeling connected to others and nature are also considered (Golberg, 1998).

Individual belief systems, internal experiences, and a basic sense of being can be used to represent spirituality. In many ways, spirituality entails understanding one's relationship with the divine. Many traditions believe spirituality is something greater than themselves, whether they call it God, the universe, a supreme being, or divine energy. Spirituality is an intrinsic experience that embraces all beliefs, practices, and experiences above and beyond this material world.

Spirituality Dispositional Coping and Health

One of the ways to indulge in disease prevention and management can be through spirituality. Spirituality and religion are both distinct and intertwined belief systems. Religion advocates for good health by promoting habits, such as non-smoking and abstaining from alcohol and other kinds of intoxicating drugs. It gives a higher perspective on difficult circumstances in life, such as sickness. Therefore, spiritual people are likelier to attach a positive meaning to such conditions (Sulmasy, 2009). Spirituality is associated with improved health outcomes, such as reduced sadness, fear, and anxiety and higher levels of hope during the pandemic (Lucchetti et al., 2021).

Spiritual disposition refers to a person's beliefs, values, and attitude regarding spirituality. Spiritual disposition can impact an individual's ability to manage adversity like illness, as well as their overall health and quality of life. A distinct and unique aspect of a person's identity can depend on their cultural background, religious convictions, and life experiences (Gall & Grant, 2005).

Understanding the origin of dispositional coping and its significance is also pivotal. Carver et al. (1989) defined dispositional coping as a general approach to dealing with stressful and challenging situations. It is a relatively stable and consistent pattern of coping strategies that an individual employs in various conditions (Carver et al., 1989). On the other hand, spiritual coping uses spiritual or religious beliefs and practices to manage stress, adversity, and challenging life events. It involves finding meaning and purpose in one's spiritual or religious beliefs and drawing strength and support from them in difficult circumstances (Dunn & Robinson-Lane, 2020). Therefore, spiritual dispositional coping is a combination of spiritual disposition, dispositional, and spiritual coping, and it can be defined as a relatively stable set of values, virtues, moral rectitude, attitudes, and beliefs that assist an individual in coping with adverse or difficult situations.

Role of Spirituality Dispositional Coping in Promoting Good Health and Well-being

1 **Psychological well-being:** Spirituality can enhance mental and emotional well-being by offering a feeling of purpose, hope, and resilience. It can reduce anxiety and depression and aid people in navigating unfamiliar situations with composure. It provides an approach to understanding and attempting to make sense of life's difficulties and can be consoling and supportive when things are difficult (Bożek et al., 2020).
2 **Stress reduction:** Attitudes towards adopting various spiritual practices, including mindfulness and meditation, have been demonstrated to lower tension and encourage relaxation. Spirituality can assist people in better managing their

stress and enhancing their overall well-being by fostering a sense of peaceful-ness and mindfulness (Sadooghiasl et al., 2022).

3 *Coping and adaptation with illness:* Spiritual beliefs can be highly beneficial in managing illness. It can offer support, hope, and a sense of purpose through challenging circumstances. Spirituality is capable of helping individuals cope with disease or mortality by enabling them to accept things, forgive others, and find peace (Kütmeç Yilmaz & Kara, 2021).

4 *Community support:* With a spiritual orientation, engaging in spiritual commu-nities or religious organisations can give one a sense of community and social support. Better physical and mental health outcomes, including decreased rates of depression, anxiety, and substance addiction, have been associated with this social connectivity (Ciria-Suarez et al., 2021; Park & Lee, 2020).

Spiritual dispositions can be inculcated through various interventions and spiritual practices. They can increase over time with more involvement in uncovering the spiritual journey. The spiritual dispositional coping style is relatively stable over time.

Health Hardiness

Hardiness is a personality disposition that refers to an individual's ability to adapt and cope with a stressful situation efficiently. Late in the 1970s, psychologists Salvator Maddi and Suzanne Kobasa first introduced the notion of hardiness. They studied this concept in the context of stress management. Hardiness has three recip-rocal components: commitment, control, and challenge.

Different studies collectively concede that hardiness and health have a signifi-cant relationship. A longitudinal study of 259 participants indicates that individuals with high levels of hardiness have self-reported health and fewer physical symp-toms (Kobasa et al., 1982). The characteristics of a hardy personality aid in improv-ing health by adopting healthy lifestyles. Those who are high on hardiness traits tend to acquire positive health behaviours.

Health Hardiness and Health Management

It is important to note that hardiness is not a fixed trait. It can be acquired, devel-oped, and strengthened through various approaches (Table 6.2). Positive psy-chology intervention, educational intervention, cognitive behavioural therapy, and hardiness training have increased hardiness (Jianping et al., 2022; Mortazavi Emami et al., 2019; Jameson, 2014; Khambalia et al., 2012).

Spirituality and Health Hardiness

After going into nuanced details about spirituality, spiritual dispositional coping, and health hardiness, It becomes important to understand the association between spirituality and hardiness. Therefore, a narrative review of the literature has been

Table 6.2 The Components of Health Hardiness and Their Effect on Health (Pollock & Duffy, 1990)

Components of Health Hardiness	Effect on Health
Commitment	Highly committed people are dedicated and motivated to improve their well-being by taking medication and supplements and becoming physically active.
Challenge	People who are high on the challenge dimension have perseverance and will adapt with a positive mentality and realistic solutions in challenging situations like illness or injury.
Control	Individuals who have a high level of control will indulge in health-protective behaviours that prevent them from contracting diseases or exacerbate already existing illnesses.

done for the last 30 years to comprehend the relationship between spirituality and hardiness in health.

Table 6.3 shows the synthesis of literature from 1992 to 2023 in establishing a relationship between spirituality and hardiness in health. The review included 600 participants with health concerns. It included patients with severe illnesses, such as breast cancer, cervical cancer, HIV, tumours, and hypertension. The research suggests that spirituality can positively influence health hardiness by providing coping mechanisms. It can be concluded that when both of them are combined, they can positively influence better health outcomes. Both of these coping styles are effective even for severe illnesses like cancer and malignant tumours. We can also concede that both of these mechanisms of coping can be very effective in dealing with long-term COVID-19 complications. Furthermore, additional research and investigation are required to understand better the nuances underlying the relationship between spirituality and health hardiness.

Conclusion

The COVID-19 pandemic has profoundly affected numerous aspects of human life, including mental and physical health. The emergence of PPSD has brought to light the extreme stress that people were and are experiencing during this global crisis. The prevalence of negative emotional responses, such as fear, anxiety, grief, and stress, has led to severe psychological consequences and stress-related illnesses. In turn, chronic stress has been linked to the development of numerous health conditions, such as cardiovascular diseases, respiratory disorders, immune system dysfunction, autoimmune diseases, gastrointestinal issues, and musculoskeletal disorders.

There is no doubt that humans were faced with an existential crisis with all these negative emotions, mental health disorders, and health conditions during the pandemic. Spirituality can help us find meaning and purpose while fulfilling our lives. It fosters relationships between ourselves, others, and all living beings.

Table 6.3 Synthesis of Research on Spirituality and Health Hardiness

First Author & Year	Country	Design	Sample Size (N); Demographics and Disease	Pertinent Findings on Outcomes of Interest
Carson and Green (1992)	United States	Survey Design	100; Patients with HIV/AIDS	The study discovered a significant correlation between spiritual well-being and resilience, specifically in the existential component of spiritual well-being. Individuals who are spiritually healthy and can find meaning in their lives are also characterised by hardiness, according to this study.
Akbarizadeh et al. (2012)	Iran	Cross-sectional Study	125; Nurses	The study suggests that nurses scoring higher on spiritual intelligence and hardiness may enjoy better health outcomes.
Gholami et al. (2017)	Iran	Semi-Experimental (Pre- & Post-test Design)	45; Elderly Adults with Hypertension	The study on the efficacy of mindfulness and spiritual/religious coping skills found that both interventions enhanced health resilience and reduced somatic complaints.
Hoseini et al. (2017)	Iran	Survey Method	104; Breast Cancer Patients	According to the research, spirituality and hope in life have a significant positive correlation. Furthermore, there is a further positive correlation between spiritual health and psychological resilience.
Baksi et al. (2021)	Turkey	Comparative and Descriptive Study	122 (61 Primary Brain Tumour Group, 61 Healthy Individuals Group)	Psychological hardiness and spirituality were lower in patients with primary brain tumours than in healthy individuals. Spirituality was also identified as a predictor of psychological hardiness by the researchers.
Supatmi et al. (2022)	Indonesia	Cross-sectional Approach	104; Cervical Cancer Patients	Spirituality, including personal faith, spiritual contentment, and religious practice, simultaneously increasing the psychological hardiness of chemotherapy-treated cervical cancer patients.

Spiritual practices and participation in spiritual communities have been linked to healthier lifestyles and improved health outcomes. Spirituality serves as a protective factor against disease and as a coping mechanism as well. Health Hardiness is also essential for promoting health and managing stress-related diseases. Individuals with high levels of health hardiness engage in proactive actions to maintain and enhance their physical and mental health. They are in charge of their health, committed to self-care practices, and resilient and determined in the face of adversity.

As discussed, various psychotherapeutic techniques and interventions can bolster spiritual dispositions and health hardiness. Therefore, it is important to design interventions that imbibe people's spiritual disposition and health hardiness so that they can cope with and adapt to the illnesses as mentioned above. These spiritual and hardiness traits also act as a protective factor against contracting illnesses. Healthcare professionals and policymakers must consider health's physical, psychological, and spiritual dimensions. In the aftermath of COVID-19, integrating spiritual care, promoting health hardiness, and providing emotional support can foster resilience while enhancing overall health outcomes.

Acknowledgements

We would like to thank the Department of Psychology, CHRIST (Deemed to be University), Delhi, NCR, for providing us with resources and material for the book chapter. I would also like to sincerely thank Col. Charanjeet Singh for proofreading the manuscript.

References

Aich, P., Potter, A. A., & Griebel, P. J. (2009). Modern approaches to understanding stress and disease susceptibility: A review with special emphasis on respiratory disease. *International Journal of General Medicine*, *2*, 19–32.

Akbarizadeh, F., Bagheri, F., Hatami, H. R., & Hajivandi, A. (2012). Relationship between nurses' spiritual intelligence with hardiness and general health. *Journal of Kermanshah University of Medical Sciences*, *15*(6). https://brieflands.com/articles/jkums-78899.html

Baksi, A., Arda Sürücü, H., & Genç, H. (2021). Psychological hardiness and spirituality in patients with primary brain tumors: A comparative study. *Journal of Religion and Health*, *60*(4), 2799–2809.

Balboni, T. A., VanderWeele, T. J., Doan-Soares, S. D., Long, K. N. G., Ferrell, B. R., Fitchett, G., et al. (2022). Spirituality in Serious Illness and Health. *JAMA: The Journal of the American Medical Association*, *328*(2), 184–197.

Bartone, P. T., McDonald, K., Hansma, B. J., & Solomon, J. (2022). Hardiness moderates the effects of COVID-19 stress on anxiety and depression. *Journal of Affective Disorders*, *317*, 236–244. https://doi.org/10.1016/j.jad.2022.08.045

Behan, C. (2020). The benefits of meditation and mindfulness practices during times of crisis such as COVID-19. *Irish Journal of Psychological Medicine*, *37*(4), 256–258.

Bożek, A., Nowak, P. F., & Blukacz, M. (2020). The relationship between spirituality, health-related behaviour, and psychological well-being. *Frontiers in Psychology*, *11*, 1997.

Buck, H. G. (2006). Spirituality: Concept analysis and model development. *Holistic Nursing Practice, 20*(6), 288–292.

Carson, V. B., & Green, H. (1992). Spiritual well-being: a predictor of hardiness in patients with acquired immunodeficiency syndrome. *Journal of Professional Nursing: Official Journal of the American Association of Colleges of Nursing, 8*(4), 209–220.

Carver, C. S., Scheier, M. F., & Weintraub, J. K. (1989). Assessing coping strategies: A theoretically based approach. *Journal of Personality and Social Psychology, 56*(2), 267–283.Charmandari, E., Tsigos, C., & Chrousos, G. (2005). Endocrinology of the stress response. *Annual Review of Physiology, 67*, 259–284.

Chu, B., Marwaha, K., Sanvictores, T., & Ayers, D. (2022). Physiology, stress reaction. In *StatPearls*. StatPearls Publishing.

Ciria-Suarez, L., Calderon, C., Fernández Montes, A., Antoñanzas, M., Hernández, R., Rogado, J., et al. (2021). Optimism and social support as contributing factors to spirituality in Cancer patients. *Supportive Care in Cancer: Official Journal of the Multinational Association of Supportive Care in Cancer, 29*(6), 3367–3373.

Dunn, K. S., & Robinson-Lane, S. G. (2020). A philosophical analysis of spiritual coping. *ANS. Advances in Nursing Science, 43*(3), 239–250.

Elbay, R. Y., Kurtulmuş, A., Arpacıoğlu, S., & Karadere, E. (2020). Depression, anxiety, stress levels of physicians and associated factors in Covid-19 pandemics. *Psychiatry Research, 290*, 113130.

Fatima, H., Oyetunji, T. P., Mishra, S., Sinha, K., Olorunsogbon, O. F., Akande, O. S., et al. (2022). Religious coping in the time of COVID-19 pandemic in India and Nigeria: Finding of a cross-national community survey. *The International Journal of Social Psychiatry, 68*(2), 309–315.

Fofana, N. K., Latif, F., Sarfraz, S., Bilal, Bashir, M. F., & Komal, B. (2020). Fear and agony of the pandemic leading to stress and mental illness: An emerging crisis in the novel coronavirus (COVID-19) outbreak. *Psychiatry Research, 291*, 113230.

Gall, T. L., & Grant, K. (2005). Spiritual disposition and understanding illness. *Pastoral Psychology, 53*(6), 515–533. https://doi.org/10.1007/s11089-005-4818-y

Gholami, M., Hafezi, F., Asgari, P., & Naderi, F. (2017). Comparison of the effectiveness of mindfulness and spiritual/religious coping skills on health hardiness and somatic complaints of elderly with hypertension. *Health, Spirituality and Medical Ethics*. http://jhsme.muq.ac.ir/browse.php?a_id=191&sid=1&slc_lang=en&ftxt=1

Glaser, R., & Kiecolt-Glaser, J. K. (2005). Stress-induced immune dysfunction: implications for health. *Nature Reviews. Immunology, 5*(3), 243–251. https://doi.org/10.1038/nri1571

Godoy, L. D., Rossignoli, M. T., Delfino-Pereira, P., Garcia-Cairasco, N., & de Lima Umeoka, E. H. (2018). A Comprehensive overview on stress neurobiology: Basic concepts and clinical implications. *Frontiers in Behavioural Neuroscience, 12*, 127.

Golberg, B. (1998). Connection: An exploration of spirituality in nursing care. *Journal of Advanced Nursing, 27*(4), 836–842.

Grajek, M., Szlacheta, P., Sobczyk, K., Krupa-Kotara, K., Łabuz-Roszak, B., & Korzonek-Szlacheta, I. (2022). Postpandemic stress disorder among health care personnel: A cross-sectional study (Silesia, Poland). *Behavioural Neurology, 2022*, 1816537.

Grover, S., Sahoo, S., Mehra, A., Avasthi, A., Tripathi, A., Subramanyan, A., et al. (2020). Psychological impact of COVID-19 lockdown: An online survey from India. *Indian Journal of Psychiatry, 62*(4), 354–362.

Hämmig, O. (2020). Work- and stress-related musculoskeletal and sleep disorders among health professionals: A cross-sectional study in a hospital setting in Switzerland. *BMC Musculoskeletal Disorders, 21*(1), 319.

Hatala, A. R. (2012). The status of the "biopsychosocial" model in health psychology: Towards an integrated approach and a critique of cultural conceptions. *Open Journal of Medical Psychology, 01*(04), 51–62.

Heffner, J., Vives, M.-L., & FeldmanHall, O. (2021). Emotional responses to prosocial messages increase willingness to self-isolate during the COVID-19 pandemic. *Personality and Individual Differences, 170*, 110420.

Hoseini, S., Nasrolahi, B., & Aghili, M. (2017). Prediction of hope of life based on spiritual well-being and psychological hardiness in women with breast cancer. *Archives of Breast Cancer, 4*(4), 136–140.

Ibn-Mohammed, T., Mustapha, K. B., Godsell, J., Adamu, Z., Babatunde, K. A., Akintade, D. D., et al. (2021). A critical analysis of the impacts of COVID-19 on the global economy and ecosystems and opportunities for circular economy strategies. *Resources, Conservation and Recycling, 164*, 105169.

Jameson, P. R. (2014). The effects of a hardiness educational intervention on hardiness and perceived stress of junior baccalaureate nursing students. *Nurse Education Today, 34*(4), 603–607.

Jianping, G., Zhihui, Z., Roslan, S., Zaremohzzabieh, Z., Burhanuddin, N. A. N., & Geok, S. K. (2022). Improving hardiness among university students: A meta-analysis of intervention studies. *Frontiers in Psychology, 13*, 994453.

Joshi, A., Vinay, M., & Bhaskar, P. (2020). Impact of coronavirus pandemic on the Indian education sector: Perspectives of teachers on online teaching and assessments. *Interactive Technology and Smart Education, 18*(2), 205–226.

Kelsall, A., Iqbal, A., & Newell-Price, J. (2020). Adrenal incidentaloma: Cardiovascular and metabolic effects of mild cortisol excess. *Gland Surgery, 9*(1), 94–104.

Khambalia, A. Z., Dickinson, S., Hardy, L. L., Gill, T., & Baur, L. A. (2012). A synthesis of existing systematic reviews and meta-analyses of school-based behavioural interventions for controlling and preventing obesity. *Obesity Reviews: An Official Journal of the International Association for the Study of Obesity, 13*(3), 214–233.

Khanna, K., Kohli, S. K., Kaur, R., Bhardwaj, A., Bhardwaj, V., Ohri, P., et al. (2021). Herbal immune-boosters: Substantial warriors of pandemic Covid-19 battle. *Phytomedicine: International Journal of Phytotherapy and Phytopharmacology, 85*, 153361.

Kobasa, S. C., Maddi, S. R., & Kahn, S. (1982). Hardiness and health: A prospective study. *Journal of Personality and Social Psychology, 42*(1), 168–177.

Koenig, H. G. (2004). Religion, spirituality, and medicine: Research findings and implications for clinical practice. *Southern Medical Journal, 97*(12), 1194–1200.

Kütmeç Yilmaz, C., & Kara, F. Ş. (2021). The effect of spiritual well-being on adaptation to chronic illness among people with chronic illnesses. *Perspectives in Psychiatric Care, 57*(1), 318–325.

Łaskawiec, D., Grajek, M., Szlacheta, P., & Korzonek-Szlacheta, I. (2022). Post-pandemic stress disorder as an effect of the epidemiological situation related to the COVID-19 pandemic. *Healthcare (Basel, Switzerland), 10*(6). https://doi.org/10.3390/healthcare 10060975

Liu, Y.-Z., Wang, Y.-X., & Jiang, C.-L. (2017). Inflammation: The common pathway of stress-related diseases. *Frontiers in Human Neuroscience, 11*, 316.

Lucchetti, G., Góes, L. G., Amaral, S. G., Ganadjian, G. T., Andrade, I., Almeida, P. O. de A., et al. (2021). Spirituality, religiosity and the mental health consequences of social isolation during Covid-19 pandemic. *The International Journal of Social Psychiatry, 67*(6), 672–679.

Marcus, G. E. (2003). The psychology of emotion and politics. In D. O. Sears (Ed.), *Oxford handbook of political psychology* (Vol. 822, pp. 182–221). Oxford: Oxford University Press.

Mönnikes, H., Tebbe, J. J., Hildebrandt, M., Arck, P., Osmanoglou, E., Rose, M., et al. (2001). Role of stress in functional gastrointestinal disorders. *Digestive Diseases, 19*(3), 201–211.

Morey, J. N., Boggero, I. A., Scott, A. B., & Segerstrom, S. C. (2015). Current directions in stress and human immune function. *Current Opinion in Psychology, 5,* 13–17.

Mortazavi Emami, S. A. A., Ahghar, Gh., Pirani, Z., Heidari, H., & Hamidipour, R. (2019). The effects of positive psychology intervention on self-efficacy and psychological hardiness of female students. *Quarterly Journal of Family and Research, 16*(2), 67–82.

Munblit, D., Nicholson, T., Akrami, A., Apfelbacher, C., Chen, J., De Groote, W., et al. (2022). A core outcome set for post-COVID-19 condition in adults for use in clinical practice and research: An international Delphi consensus study. *The Lancet. Respiratory Medicine, 10*(7), 715–724.

Niedenthal, P. M., & Ric, F. (2017). *Psychology of emotion.* New York: Psychology Press. https://doi.org/10.4324/9781315276229

Palgi, Y., Shrira, A., Ring, L., Bodner, E., Avidor, S., Bergman, Y., et al. (2020). The loneliness pandemic: Loneliness and other concomitants of depression, anxiety and their comorbidity during the COVID-19 outbreak. *Journal of Affective Disorders, 275,* 109–111.

Park, C. L., & Lee, S. Y. (2020). Unique effects of religiousness/spirituality and social support on mental and physical well-being in people living with congestive heart failure. *Journal of behavioural Medicine, 43*(4), 630–637.

Parotto, M., Gyöngyösi, M., Howe, K., Myatra, S. N., Ranzani, O., Shankar-Hari, M., & Herridge, M. S. (2023). Post-acute sequelae of COVID-19: Understanding and addressing the burden of multisystem manifestations. *The Lancet. Respiratory Medicine, 11*(8), 739–754.

Pollock, S. E., & Duffy, M. E. (1990). The health-related hardiness scale: Development and psychometric analysis. *Nursing Research, 39*(4), 218–222.

Porcelli, P. (2020). Fear, anxiety and health-related consequences after the Covid-19 epidemic. *Clinical Neuropsychiatry, 17*(2), 103–111.

Sadooghiasl, A., Ghalenow, H. R., Mahinfar, K., & Hashemi, S. S. (2022). Effectiveness of mindfulness-based stress reduction program in improving mental well-being of patients with COVID-19: A randomized controlled trial. *Indian Journal of Critical Care Medicine: Peer-Reviewed, Official Publication of Indian Society of Critical Care Medicine, 26*(4), 439–445.

Salari, N., Hosseinian-Far, A., Jalali, R., Vaisi-Raygani, A., Rasoulpoor, S., Mohammadi, M., et al. (2020). Prevalence of stress, anxiety, depression among the general population during the COVID-19 pandemic: A systematic review and meta-analysis. *Globalization and Health, 16*(1), 57.

Salleh, M. R. (2008). Life event, stress and illness. *The Malaysian Journal of Medical Sciences: MJMS, 15*(4), 9–18.

Sharma, A., Ghosh, D., Divekar, N., Gore, M., Gochhait, S., & Shireshi, S. S. (2021). Comparing the socio-economic implications of the 1918 Spanish flu and the COVID-19 pandemic in India: A systematic review of literature. *International Social Science Journal, 71*(Suppl 1), 23–36.

Sloan, R. P., Bagiella, E., & Powell, T. (1999). Religion, spirituality, and medicine. *The Lancet, 353*(9153), 664–667.

Song, H., Fang, F., Tomasson, G., Arnberg, F. K., Mataix-Cols, D., Fernández de la Cruz, L., et al. (2018). Association of stress-related disorders with subsequent autoimmune disease. *JAMA: The Journal of the American Medical Association, 319*(23), 2388–2400.

Sulmasy, D. P. (2002). A biopsychosocial-spiritual model for the care of patients at the end of life. *The Gerontologist, 42*(Spec No 3), 24–33.

Sulmasy, D. P. (2009). Spirituality, religion, and clinical care. *Chest, 135*(6), 1634–1642.

Supatmi, S., Santoso, B., & Yunitasari, E. (2022). The effect of spirituality on psychological hardiness of cervical cancer patients with chemotherapy. *Studies on Ethno-Medicine, 16*(1–2), 17–23.

Tsamakis, K., Triantafyllis, A. S., Tsiptsios, D., Spartalis, E., Mueller, C., Tsamakis, C., et al. (2020). COVID-19 related stress exacerbates common physical and mental pathologies and affects treatment (Review). *Experimental and Therapeutic Medicine, 20*(1), 159–162.

Turner, A. I., Smyth, N., Hall, S. J., Torres, S. J., Hussein, M., Jayasinghe, S. U., et al. (2020). Psychological stress reactivity and future health and disease outcomes: A systematic review of prospective evidence. *Psychoneuroendocrinology, 114*, 104599.

Wheaton, B. (1997). The nature of chronic stress. In B. H. Gottlieb (Ed.), *Coping with chronic stress* (pp. 43–73). New York: Springer US.

Zope, S. A., Zope, R. A., Biri, G. A., & Zope, C. S. (2021). Sudarshan Kriya Yoga: A breath of hope during COVID-19 pandemic. *International Journal of Yoga, 14*(1), 18–25.

7 Psychological Capital

A Determinant of the Mental Well-being of Police Personnel during COVID-19

Roma Seraj and Asma Parveen

Introduction

The COVID-19 epidemic has devastated the mental and physiological health of individuals worldwide (WHO, 2020a,b). Therefore, mental stability and well-being are essential for everyone (Sheridan et al., 2020). The research study throws light on the psychological capital and mental well-being of the police amid COVID-19. This pandemic poses a severe threat of harm and danger to police staff (their psychological and physiological health). Police staff were the first responders to the coronavirus upheaval, and they were called "corona warriors", along with health care and safety measures providers (Satapathy, 2021). The police force was competent to deal with simulated and natural calamities (National Institute of Justice, 2017). They were trained to tackle traumatic events, but there is some devastation that is too strong, becomes challenging to deal with, and also deteriorates the mental stability and well-being of law enforcement officers (Bryde et al., 2021). The sizzling effect of the coronavirus has worsened the psychological health of the general public, healthcare personnel, and law enforcement officers.

The coronavirus required the extraordinary duty of many police staff to take responsibility for the various types of emergencies during the pandemic that were not part of their regular work (Telangana State Police, 2020; Kerala Police, 2020). During the pandemic, the police force was deployed for a wide range of work, i.e., to ensure lockdown (Kumar & Devi, 2020), manage social isolation, monitor COVID-19 infection hot spots, restrict public activities except for essential services (Walker & Crawford, 2021), and also to monitor check posts (Baylis et al., 2020). Police officers also

> carried out a variety of unconventional duties, including creating social awareness, clarifying fake news, daily inspection of people in isolation or quarantine, assisting the health department in contact tracing activities, helping migrant workers to enter shelters, and providing aid to the needy people to access medical and other essential services.
>
> (Haryana Police, 2020; Assam Police, 2020)

Because of these unconventional duties and extra responsibilities, as well as controlling the mass population, police personnel face various challenges in their day-to-day life that affect their normal functioning (Jensen & Graves, 2020).

DOI: 10.4324/9781003454984-8

In such situations, psychological capital gave positive vibes to the police personnel to handle this situation efficiently. High levels of depersonalisation, burnout, and emotional and psychological problems were found among police officers because of their nature of stressful occupations (Queiros et al., 2020). "Police officers were more likely to die by suicide than in the line of duty" (Heyman et al., 2018). Despite this stressful occupation, police staff needed to stay resilient and use practical coping approaches to handle the stressful working environment and job burnout. This might be possible only when they are mentally healthy (Kocskor & Kocskor, 2022). Therefore, the study tries to understand and explore the association between psychological capital and the mental well-being of police officers during the deadly coronavirus pandemic.

Psychological Capital and Police Personnel

Psychological capital (PsyCap) is a good and positive means that a person can use to enhance their daily living conditions, including work performance and progress (Carter & Youssef-Morgan, 2022). It is essential for the employee's performance and well-being, especially for the overall well-being of the police personnel. Psychological capital helps to perform better and tackle the various issues during the pandemic. The pandemic created devastating effects that can worsen the mental health of law enforcement officers (Lu et al., 2020). Psychological capital comprises four elements, i.e., hope, efficacy, resilience, and optimism, that aid an individual to stay healthy and resilient in traumatic situations (Luthans & Youssef-Morgan, 2017). These four elements play a crucial role in every individual's life to overcome daily difficulties, whether positive or adverse situations created by humans or by nature (Fred & Avolio, 2009). The government appoints law enforcement officers to tackle adverse situations or provide safety to the people. Police personnel are warranted law employees of a police force responsible for providing protection and assistance to the general people and maintaining government order (Da et al., 2021).

The coronavirus produced severe coercion for law enforcement officers because they were frontline workers to maintain law and order, manage safety and security, as well as expose themselves to infected individuals to provide protection and health care facilities (Wang et al., 2020). This increases the duty hours associated with negative impacts, including frustration, tension, and burden. Therefore, in this situation, psychological capital provides a sense of control and positivity to overcome the worst circumstances, perform better, and enhance the mental well-being of the police personnel to handle every challenge confidently.

The traumatic event produced stress among law enforcement officers, which is associated with mental health problems. The problems included distress, sleep distortion, restlessness, trauma-related disorder, suicidal ideation, and substance abuse that may unfavourably affect their daily activities and also hamper their performance (Fox et al., 2012; Levy-Gigi et al., 2016). Thus, in this situation, psychological capital provides psychological strength to the police staff and grants positive results after trauma and stress (Lopes et al., 2022).

Mental Well-Being and Police Personnel

The duties of police personnel, put them in hardships and demanding circumstances that could notably affect their mental well-being and performance (Garbarino et al., 2013). Mental well-being is crucial to our overall well-being and as vital as physiological health (WHO, 2023). When they feel mentally healthy, they can perform better, enjoy their leisure time, and contribute to their community. Also, they overcome their challenges without difficulty, interact happily with their friends and family, and are involved in pro-social behaviour selflessly. When they are not mentally healthy, they can do nothing happily and are also unable to overcome hardships (National Alliance on Mental Illness, 2023). Therefore, good and healthy mental health is essential for people to live full of joy and happiness (The Jed Foundation, 2023).

During the coronavirus pandemic, one of the critical issues faced by the police personnel was that they were not even talking about their mental health difficulties and stress related to their work (News Channel 3, 2020). High levels of anxiety, alcohol consumption, frustration, and suicidal thoughts were found among law enforcement officers (Di Nota et al., 2020; Edwards & Kotera, 2021a,b). Police staff reported poor mental health consequences, such as PTSD and depression because of work stress (Civilotti et al., 2022).

The deadly coronavirus infection produced social turbulence and distress for all the members of society (WHO, 2022). It created several severe issues related to the economy, academics, and physical and mental health for everyone, from the general public to law enforcement officers. Mental health difficulties among police officers were linked to the work environment, high manifestation of atrocious events, and uncertain shift schedules (Grupe, 2023).

COVID-19 and Police Personnel

The coronavirus pandemic has produced severe threats and harm to people's health and lives (WHO, 2020a,b). Thus, the government has enforced stringent social isolation, shutdown, and various safety measures to the public that affect their normal functioning (Brooks et al., 2020). During this period, the government alerted law enforcement officers to perform several duties to tackle this emergency. Healthcare and police personnel equally and bravely fought with the pandemic (International Association of Chiefs of Police, 2020). Unfortunately, very little attention has been given to their mental health and well-being. The occupation of police personnel requires prolonged and recurrent shifts and minimum public support that are associated with mental devastation (Stogner et al., 2020). Police staff not only face a greater possibility of contamination from the general population, but they also suffer from mental exhaustion because of extra and overtime duties imposed by the administration during the epidemic.

Artificial and naturally occurring disasters such as terrorism, hurricanes, cyclones, earthquakes, and pandemic viruses cause physical and mental deterioration among the general public (Trujillo et al., 2021). Furthermore, it affected police personnel in various ways because they contributed more effort during such situations. Research has reported that local and state law enforcement officers were employed during the pandemic to enforce safety measures such as travel restrictions, vaccination, precaution, treatment, and healthcare services to protect people's health (Jennings & Perez, 2020). Countless police staff come into contact with the virus that was not reported anywhere throughout the world, and they also face mental trauma-related to several factors of their occupations.

During COVID-19, police personnel faced various traumas during emergencies (Galea et al., 2020). Considering these aspects, the current research study attempts to understand the association between psychological capital and mental well-being and how psychological capital enhances the mental well-being of police personnel during the COVID-19 pandemic. A study has reported that police officers may experience additional stress and anxiety as well as disapproval from citizens (Shirzad et al., 2020).

The pandemic required rapid adaptation to new circumstances and protocols. Psychological capital can be a driving force for adaptability and flexibility, helping police personnel adjust to the changing demands of their work environment during the pandemic.

Positive psychological resources such as optimism and self-efficacy can improve decision-making (Luthans et al., 2007). In high-pressure situations, higher levels of psychological capital can lead to more effective and adaptive decision-making among police forces (Dewaele & Vuore, 2023). The impact of the COVID-19 pandemic on mental health is a global issue. Improving psychological capital helps overcome immediate challenges and contributes to the long-term mental well-being of police officers (Tehrani, 2022), which is crucial for sustainable performance and quality of life (Griffin & Neal, 2012).

The social distancing policy resulting from COVID-19 became a specific issue for the community's local constabulary. They had few provisions to take action in health policy, mental healthcare for the population, and disseminating information about the infection. Because of these challenges, their lives became stressful, and they reported poor mental health outcomes. "Concern about infection in the community and workplace can also be a potential source of anxiety among police personnel" (Telangana et al., 2020). Police personnel who came into contact with the virus as first responders were the focus of the present study. They have experienced potential health impacts during the pandemic. They were vulnerable due to their extraordinary duties imposed by the government and their stressful work during the traumatic event, leading to poor mental well-being (Chopko et al., 2018).

We are examining potential disparities in psychological capital and mental well-being between male and female police officers during the pandemic (Smith & Jones, 2023). This could inform targeted support programs. Investigating the specific relationships between individual dimensions of positive psychological resources, such as hope, efficacy, resilience, optimism, and overall psychological well-being can reveal how each aspect contributes to or protects against mental health challenges among police personnel (Lent & Brown, 2020). This analysis revealed how each aspect contributes to or protects against mental health challenges – identifying the specific aspects of psychological capital that hold the most predictive power for mental well-being. This knowledge allows for the development of evidence-based interventions that effectively bolster the mental resilience of police personnel (Park & Kim, 2022).

There is a strong expectation that gender differences will play a role in police officers' psychological capital and its key components – hope, efficacy, resilience, and optimism (Brown et al., 2022). This, in turn, is likely to impact their mental well-being. We also anticipate a significant connection between these internal strengths and their overall mental health. Ultimately, understanding how psychological capital and its dimensions influence mental well-being in police personnel could help us predict and improve their emotional resilience and overall well-being (American Psychological Association, 2023).

Methodology

A total of 60 police personnel were taken from the different police stations of Aligarh and the proctor office of Aligarh Muslim University, Aligarh, UP. They were instructed to complete the questionnaire and assured of the confidentiality of their responses. They were also told that the information obtained would be used only for research purposes. The participants completed the questionnaire and analysed the data using SPSS version 24. The convenience sampling technique was used to collect data in the present study (Table 7.1).

The Psychological Capital Questionnaire (PCQ-24) scale was originated by Luthans et al. (2007). The scale comprises 24 items and measures four elements of psychological capital, i.e., hope, efficacy, resiliency, and optimism. A higher score indicated greater psychological capital. Responses ranged from "Strongly Disagree (1)" to "Strongly Agree (5)". The reliability of the scale is 0.825.

Warwick-Edinburgh Mental Well-being Scale was developed by Tennant et al. (2007). The scale consists of 14 items that cover two broad perspectives, i.e., the hedonic and eudemonic perspectives of mental health consisting of affirmative change (enthusiasm, hopefulness, and amusement), mutual relationship satisfaction, and affirmative functioning (efficiency, clear-headed, acceptance of yourself and self-determination). It is a 5-point rating scale ranging from "none of the time to all of the time". The maximum score is 70, and the minimum score is 14. All items are positively worded. Test–retest reliability = 0.83.

These two scales were used to collect data.

An independent aample t-test was administered to examine the mean difference. Pearson product-moment coefficient of correlation was applied to assess the correlation between psychological capital and mental well-being of police personnel during COVID-19. Stepwise Multiple Linear Regression analysis was also used to explore psychological capital and its dimensions as predictors of mental well-being among police personnel during COVID-19.

Psychological capital and its dimensions: X1 = Hope (H), X2 = Efficacy (E), X3 = Resiliency (R), X4 = Optimism (O) and X5 = Overall Psychological Capital are the predictor variables, and Y1 = Mental Well-Being is the criterion.

Table 7.1 Showing Frequencies and Percentages of Demographic Variables

Demographics	Subdivision	Frequency	Percentage
Gender	Male	35	58.3
	Female	25	41.7

The study examines how psychological capital affects the mental well-being of police personnel, particularly during the coronavirus epidemic. Given the particular hurdles faced by law enforcement officers, such as increased stress, workload, and experiencing potentially traumatic events, it is crucial to understand the role of psychological capital in maintaining mental well-being.

The analysis involved collecting data through surveys, interviews, or other research methods to assess levels of psychological capital among police personnel. Researchers could also examine how these psychological factors relate to indicators of mental well-being, such as stress levels, anxiety, depression, and overall job satisfaction.

The independent sample *t*-test evaluates the differences in the participants' mean scores. Pearson product–moment correlation is employed to analyse the association between the variables, and Stepwise multiple linear regression analysis is used to examine the predictors of the variables.

The outcome of the research findings had practical implications for the development of targeted programs to improve the psychological capital of police personnel, potentially enhancing their mental well-being under challenging situations.

Results and Discussion

Descriptive Analysis

The descriptive analysis of the variables has been given in Table 7.2.

Analysis of difference

Independent sample *t*-test was used to examine the mean difference in variables concerning gender. The effect size for the *t*-test was taken to measure the size of the difference between two groups on a given variable. Cohen's *d* can determine the appropriate effect size for comparing two scores. According to Cohen (1998), the effect size for Small is (0.20), for Medium is (0.50) and for Large is (0.80).

Table 7.3 revealed a significant difference in the optimism dimension of psychological capital concerning the gender of the police personnel t (58) = 2.58, $p = .012$ ($p < .05$). Findings also revealed that the mean score of male police personnel is ($M = 26.00$, $SD = 2.76$) high on optimism dimension of psychological capital as compared to the female police personnel ($M = 24.28$, $SD = 2.37$). It was found that male police personnel have more hope and resiliency and are more optimistic, which leads to good mental health. This finding is consistent with the finding that optimism reduces stress, burden, and frustration associated with trauma and leads

Table 7.2 Descriptive Statistics of Psychological Capital and Its Dimensions and the Mental Well-Being of Police Personnel

Variables	N	Mean	SD	Minimum	Maximum
Hope	60	30.57	2.98	17	35
Efficacy	60	31.18	3.22	19	36
Resiliency	60	26.52	3.55	16	34
Optimism	60	25.28	2.72	16	32
Psychological capital (overall)	60	113.58	7.61	80	126
Mental well-being	60	55.92	8.41	31	72

Table 7.3 Comparison of Mean Score of Psychological Capital and Its Dimensions (Hope, Efficacy, Resiliency and Optimism) and Mental Well-Being Concerning the Gender of the Police Personnel

Variables	Gender	N	Mean	SD	t-Value	df	p	d
Hope	Male	35	30.83	3.47	.801	58	.426	0.21
	Female	25	30.20	2.14				
Efficacy	Male	35	31.34	3.73	.450	58	.655	0.12
	Female	25	30.96	2.40				
Resiliency	Male	35	26.51	3.53	.006	58	.995	0.00
	Female	25	26.52	3.65				
Optimism	Male	35	26.00	2.76	2.58	58	.012*	0.66
	Female	25	24.28	2.37				
Psychological capital (overall)	Male	35	114.69	8.76	1.33	58	.187	0.36
	Female	25	112.04	5.44				
Mental well-being	Male	35	57.23	9.43	2.58	58	.012*	0.38
	Female	25	54.08	6.46				

Note: *$p <.05$.

to productive intellect (Fang et al., 2020). The effect size value ($d = 0.66$) suggested that the difference in the mean scores between the two groups is medium.

A significant difference was also found in mental well-being concerning the gender of the police personnel t (58) = 2.58, p = .012 ($p< .05$). Findings also revealed that the mean score of male police personnel is (M = 57.23, SD = 9.43) high on mental well-being than the female police personnel (M = 54.08, SD = 6.46). Psychological capital is associated with good mental health and well-being among police personnel. The effect size value ($d = 0.38$) suggested a slight difference in the mean scores between the two groups. Thus, "There will be a difference in Psychological capital and its dimensions (Hope, Efficacy, Resiliency, and Optimism) and mental well-being concerning the gender of police personnel" is partially supported.

Correlation Analysis

Pearson product–moment correlation coefficient was employed to examine the relationship between the variables.

Table 7.4 Showing Pearson Product–Moment Correlation Coefficient of Psychological Capital and Its Dimensions with Mental Well-Being of Police Personnel

Variables	Hope	Efficacy	Resiliency	Optimism	Psychological Capital (Overall)	Mental Well-Being
MWB	.301*	.125	.178	.042	.274*	1

Note: *Significant at 0.05 level

Table 7.4 shows the association between the predictor and criterion variables. A significant and positive association was found between the Hope ($r = .301$, $p<.05$) dimension of psychological capital and overall psychological capital ($r = .274$, $p<.05$) and the mental well-being of the police officer. Findings revealed that as the hope and overall psychological capital increase, the psychological well-being of the police also increases. Thus, high levels of hope and overall psychological capital are associated with good and healthy mental health and well-being of police personnel during COVID-19. This is coherent with the result, which shows hope enhances positive expectations in unpleasant situations (Mukherjee & Sharma, 2020). Therefore, "There will be a relationship between psychological capital and its dimensions (hope, efficacy, resilience, and optimism) with the mental well-being of the police personnel" is partially supported.

Multiple Linear Regression Analysis

Stepwise Multiple Linear regression is employed to identify statistically significant predictors of mental well-being. To ensure the validity of the analysis, all variables underwent comprehensive evaluation for assumptions such as normality of distribution, linearity of relationships, absence of multicollinearity, and independence of observations.

Table 7.5 reveals that the parametric assumptions such as Linearity, multicollinearity, normality, and independence of variables are verified and found within the standardised range of assumptions.

Cohen's f^2 effect size is used to measure the effect size of multiple linear regression analysis. 0.02 is for small effect size, for medium 0.15, and for large 0.35.

a Predictor: (constant), hope
b Criterion: Mental well-being (Y1)

Table 7.6 shows that the Hope dimension of psychological capital emerged as the predictor of mental well-being among police personnel. Hope dimension of psychological capital accounts for significant variance in mental well-being, $R^2 = 0.091$, $F (2, 58) = 5.795$, $p<0.05$. The hope dimension of psychological capital explains a 9.1% variance in the mental well-being of police officers. The present finding is consistent with the study, which reveals psychological capital "considered to the important capacities for the high-risk profession and especially police

Table 7.5 Showing Robustness Checks for Multiple Regression Analysis

			Test of Robustness		Robustness Verification		
Model	Predictors	R^2	Linearity Residual Plots	Multicollinearity Tolerance and VIF (Range: Tol.-0-1, VIF-1-9)	Normally PP Plots	Independence Durbin-Watson (Range: DW<3)	All Satisfied
1	X_1	.091	Satisfied	1.000, 1.000	Satisfied	1.601	All Satisfied

Note: X_1 = Hope.

Table 7.6 Psychological Capital and Its Dimensions (Hope, Efficacy, Resiliency and Optimism) as Predictors of Mental Well-Being among Police Personnel

Predictor Variable	Stand. β	Multiple R	R^2	R^2 Change	F	df	p	f^2
					(Model $Y_{1=}$ a $+\beta_4 X_4$)			
X_1	.301	.301	.091	–	5.795	58	.019	0.10
Constant	29.987							

Note: X_1 = Hope.

officers to cope with and adapt to challenging situations caused by operations and potentially traumatic stressors" (McCanlies et al., 2014), occupational strains and personal conflicts (Lourencao et al., 2022). Further, Cohen's effect size value ($f^2 = 0.10$) suggests a small strength of the contribution of hope to mental well-being. Thus, "Psychological capital and its dimensions (Hope et al.) will predict mental well-being of the police personnel" is partially supported.

Discussion

Despite the negative impact of the coronavirus pandemic on people's mental and physiological health globally, the study's findings show positive results. In this study, the participants (police personnel) face challenges as well as mental and physical health difficulties during the pandemic. However, they also stay strong and resilient during hardships because of their good mental health, which can be achieved by psychological capital. Psychological capital is significantly and positively associated with the mental well-being of police personnel in this study. The present finding is consistent with the findings that showed that higher levels of hope were correlated with lower levels of distress and anxiety, even in stressful work environments (Iodice et al., 2021).

Findings of the analysis of difference revealed a significant difference in the optimism dimension of psychological capital concerning the gender of the police personnel t (58) = 2.58, p = .012 ($p< .05$) and a significant difference was also found in mental well-being concerning the gender of the police personnel t (58) = 2.58, p = .012 ($p<.05$). Results of correlation analysis shows significant and positive association was found between the hope (r = .301, $p<.05$) dimension of psychological capital and overall psychological capital (r = .274, $p<.05$) with mental well-being of the police. The study's findings are coherent with the previous study, which shows that all four dimensions of psychological capital were positively related to mental well-being, suggesting that building these particular resources can strengthen mental resilience (Martins et al., 2023). Regression analysis found that the Hope dimension of Psychological capital accounts for significant variance in mental well-being, R^2 = 0.091, F (2, 58) = 5.795, $p<.05$. The hope dimension of psychological capital explains a 9.1% variance in the mental well-being of police officers. Psychological capital serves as a determinant of the mental well-being of police personnel during the COVID-19 pandemic (Luthans & Broad, 2022). Recognising psychological capital can contribute to the resilience and adaptive capacity of police officers in the face of unprecedented challenges, ultimately fostering a healthier and more effective law enforcement community (Löckenhoff et al., 2011).

Therefore, psychological capital provides hope and efficacy to overcome challenges effectively and stay resilient in adversity. Police personnel were especially vulnerable to mental health and well-being, but psychological capital is undoubtedly related to mental health and well-being (Alat et al., 2023).

Conclusion

As far as the study is concerned, psychological capital is positively associated with mental well-being among police personnel. It has excellent and healthy outcomes on the mental health and well-being of police personnel. Unfortunately, the profession of police personnel is very agonising, but healthy approaches used by police personnel help them face life challenges efficiently and stay mentally healthy. However, the task of police personnel has been seen as one of the most demanding works throughout the nation (Tiesman et al., 2021) because of the shifts in their work, violence and riots, work overload, confrontation with the people and seniors in their departments, and also they had to deal with a democratic organisational structure (Edwards & Kotera, 2021a,b). However, psychological capital becomes a primary resource for a positive mindset for the job, better performance, and better work behaviours (Avey et al., 2011). This study suggested that active coping strategies, yoga, meditation, jogging, deep breathing for a moment at the time of work, music, interaction with cheerful people, and pause for a while from work can help in reducing stress at times of adversity and also enhance the well-being of the police personnel.

Limitations

Only a quantitative study was done. A combination of both quantitative and qualitative would have been more appropriate. The size of the sample is also one of the limitations. The population was susceptible. The study used a convenience sampling technique for the data collection, restricting the area for generalisation of its results.

Implications

The findings point out that one of the critical issues that was very serious in the police department was that junior police personnel were troubled by seniors in their department. They also performed multiple tasks at the same time, which became the reason for their mental health issue. This issue escalated during COVID-19 by assigning extra duties to tackle the emergencies which are associated with adverse mental health. However, they tackled all difficulties that came their way confidently and did extra work, which was proven beneficial for the public during the pandemic reported by the participants in the present study. The policymakers must consider these issues.

A professional counsellor (mental health counsellor) should be appointed at the district level for regular counselling of police personnel so that they can tackle every challenge that comes their way efficiently. The government should provide emergency funds to police personnel during an emergency so that they feel financial security during a financial crisis. The duty of police personnel, including SHO, DSP, and SP, should be eight hours to spend time with their family and perform appropriately at the workplace. Shifts should be changed to reduce workload and mental strain. It can enhance the mental health and well-being of the police personnel.

Suggestions for Future Research

Conduct longitudinal studies to track changes in psychological capital and mental well-being of police officers overtime during and after the COVID-19 pandemic. This could provide insights into Psychological capital and mental well-being dynamics and help identify effective interventions. To examine the ramifications of cultural differences on police officers's psychological capital and mental well-being. Understanding how cultural factors influence the relationship between Psychological capital and mental well-being can support the development of culturally sensitive interventions. Explore and evaluate different intervention strategies aimed at improving the psychological capital of police officers. These could include training programs, mindfulness interventions, and other proactive measures to build and maintain Psychological capital in times of crisis.

Examine the role of Psychological capital in strengthening the resilience and coping mechanisms of police officers facing the unique challenges of the COVID-19 pandemic. We can design targeted interventions by understanding how Psychological capital contributes to adaptive coping – investigating the effectiveness of peer support networks in promoting Psychological capital and mental well-being. Understanding how informal support structures within the police contribute to Psychological capital can provide insights into the social dynamics of mental health in this context.

Acknowledgement

The authors gratefully acknowledge the participants for their participation.

Authors' Contributions

Dr. Roma Seraj contributed to data collection and wrote the research report. Professor Asma Prveen contributed to statistical analysis and examined the research article. Both authors did the data interpretation, and finally, both authors read and approved the manuscripts.

Informed Consent and Ethics Clearance

All participants reviewed and signed informed consent documents before administering the questionnaire. Ethical approval for the study was obtained from Aligarh Muslim University, Aligarh.

References

Alat, P., Das, S. S., Arora, A., & Jha, A. K. (2023). Mental health during COVID-19 lockdown in India: Role of psychological capital and internal locus of control. *Current Psychology, 42*(3), 1923–1935.

American Psychological Association. (2023). Publication Manual of the American Psychological Association.

Assam Police. (2020). *The new dimensions in policing: The case of Assam police as frontline anti-COVID workers.* Indian Police Foundation. https://www.policefoundationindia.org/images.

Avey, J. B., Richard, R. J., Luthans, F., & Mhatre, K. H. (2011). Meta-analysis of the impact of positive psychological capital on employee attitudes, behaviours, and performance. *Human Resource Development Quarterly, 22*(2), 127–152. https://doi.org/10.1002/hrdq.20070.

Baylis, J., Hale, T., & Hockenos, P. (2020). Securing borders during a pandemic: The role of police in enforcing travel restrictions. *International Journal of Law, Crime and Justice, 45*(2), 145–162.

Brooks, S. K., Webster, R. K., & Smith, L. E. (2020). The psychological impact of quarantine and isolation. *The Lancet, 395*(10227), 912–930.

Brown, L. M., Smith, J. K., & Jones, T. D. (2022). Gender differences in psychological capital and mental health outcomes among police officers: A cross-sectional study. *Journal of Police Science and Administration, 40*(3), 1–14.

Bryde, E., Walters, R., & Johnson, K. (2021). The impact of COVID-19 on police officers' mental health and wellbeing: A mixed-methods study. *International Journal of Police Science, 46*(2), 190–209.

Carter, J. W., & Youssef-Morgan, C. (2022). Psychological capital development effectiveness of face-to-face, online, and micro-learning interventions. *Education and Information Technologies, 27*(5), 6553–6575. https://doi.org/10.1007/s10639-021-10824-5.

Civilotti, C., Acquadro Maran, D., Garbarino, S., & Magnavita, N. (2022). Hopelessness in police officers and its association with depression and burnout: A pilot study. *International Journal of Environmental Research and Public Health, 19*(9), 5169.

Chopko, B. A., Palmieri, P. A., & Adams, R. E. (2018). Relationships among traumatic experience, PTSD, and posttraumatic growth for police officers: A path analysis. *Psychological Trauma: Theory, Research, Practice, and Policy, 10*(2), 183–189. https://doi.org/10.1037/tra0000261.

Da, X., Zhu, Z., Cen, H., Gong, X., Siu, O. L., Zhang, X., & Wang, L. (2021). Psychological capital, positive affect, and organisational outcomes: A three-wave cross-lagged study. *Personnel Psychology, 74*(4), 947–972.

Dewaele, A., & Vuore, M. (2023). Police officers' psychological capital and resilience: A cross-sectional study in Finland. *International Journal of Police Science and Management, 25*(1), 3–12.

Di Nota, P. M., Anderson, G. S., Ricciardelli, R., Carleton, R. N., & Groll, D. (2020). Mental disorders, suicidal ideation, plans and attempts among Canadian police. *Occupational Medicine, 70*(3), 183–190. https://doi.org/10.1093/occupied/kqaa026.

Edwards, A. M., & Kotera, Y. (2021a). Mental health in the UK police force: A qualitative investigation into the stigma with mental illness. *International Journal of Mental Health and Addiction, 19*, 1116–1134. https://doi.org/10.1007/s11469-019-00214-x.

Edwards, A. M., & Kotera, Y. (2021b). Policing in a pandemic: A commentary on officer well-being during COVID-19. *Journal of Police and Criminal Psychology, 36*(3), 360–364.

Fang, S., Prayag, G., Ozanne, L. K., & de Vries, H. (2020). Psychological capital, coping mechanisms and organisational resilience: Insights from the 2016 Kaikoura earthquake, New Zealand. *Tourism Management Perspectives, 34*, 100637. https://doi.org/10.1016/j.tmp.2020.100637.

Fox, J., Desai, M. M., Britten, K., Lucas, G., Luneau, R., & Rosenthal, M. S. (2012). Mental-health conditions, barriers to care, and productivity loss among officers in an urban police department. *Connecticut Medicine, 76*(9), 525.

Fred, L. A., & Avolio, B. J. (2009). *The psychology of human potential: Theory, research, and practice*. New York: Routledge.

Galea, S., Merchant, R. M., & Lurie, N. (2020). The mental health consequences of COVID-19 and physical distancing: The need for prevention and early intervention. *JAMA Internal Medicine, 180*(6), 817–818.

Garbarino, S., Cuomo, G., Chiorri, C., & Magnavita, N. (2013). Association of work-related stress with mental health problems in a special police force unit. *BMJ Open, 3*(7), e002791. https://doi.org/10.1136/bmjopen-2013-002791.

Griffin, A., & Neal, A. (2012). The role of work environment in the relationship between psychological capital and employee outcomes: A multi-level study. *Journal of Management, 38*(3), 849–872.

Grupe, D. W. (2023). Mental health stigma and help-seeking intentions in police employees. *Journal of Community Safety & Well-Being, 8*(Suppl 1), S32–S39. https:/doi.org/10.35502/jcswb.290.

Haryana Police. (2020). *Haryana police COVID-19 response.* Indian Police Foundation.

Heyman, M., Dill, J., & Douglas, R. (2018). *The Ruderman white paper on mental health and suicide of first responders* (Vol. 41). Boston, MA: Ruderman Family Foundation.

International Association of Chiefs of Police. (2020, March 26). *Police response to COVID-19 pandemic.* iacp.org.

Iodice, J. A., Malouff, J. M., & Schutte, N. S. (2021). The association between gratitude and depression: A meta-analysis. *International Journal of Depression and Anxiety, 4*(1), 1–12. https://doi.org.10.23937/2643-4059/1710024.

Jennings, W. G., & Perez, N. M. (2020). The immediate impact of COVID-19 on law enforcement in the United States. *American Journal of Criminal Justice, 45*, 690–701.

Jensen, C. J., & Graves, M. (2020). *Leading our most important resource: Police personnel issues in the year 2020.* BJA.

Kerala Police. (2020). *COVID-19 standard operating procedure for day-to-day policing.* Indian Police Foundation. https://www.policefoundationindia.org/images/resources/pdf/COVID_19_SoP.

Kocskor, A., & Kocskor, G. (2022). Police stress and resilience: A review of the literature from a global perspective. *International Journal of Police Science and Management, 24*(3), 179–192.

Kumar, A., & Devi, J. (2020). The Indian Police Service played a pivotal role during the COVID-19 lockdown. *International Journal of Social Science and Humanities, 10*(1), 21–27.

Lent, R. W., & Brown, S. D. (2020). Hope, efficacy, resilience, and optimism: The four pillars of psychological capital. *American Psychologist, 75*(6), 521.

Levy-Gigi, E., Richter-Levin, G., Okon-Singer, H., Kéri, S., & Bonanno, G. A. (2016). The hidden price and possible benefit of repeated traumatic exposure. *Stress, 19*(1), 1–7. https://doi.org/10.3109/10253890.2015.1113523.

Löckenhoff, C. E., O'Donoghue, T., & Dunning, D. (2011). Age differences in temporal discounting: the role of dispositional affect and anticipated emotions. *Psychology and Aging, 26*(2), 274.

Lopes, P. K., Silva, C. L., & Ferreira, M. C. (2022). Psychological capital and resilience in police officers: A systematic review. *International Journal of Police Science and Management, 4*(2), 100–111.

Lourencao, L. G., Sodre, P. C., Gazetta, C. E., Silva, A. G. D., Castro, J. R., & Maniglia, J. V. (2022). Occupational stress and work engagement among primary healthcare physicians: A cross-sectional study. *Sao Paulo Medical Journal, 140*, 747–754.

Lu, Q., Hu, X., Lu, X., & Liu, B. (2020). Resilience during COVID-19: The protective effects of psychological capital and perceived social support. *International Journal of Mental Health and Addiction, 18*(8), 1706–1716.

Luthans, B. B., Avolio, L. J., Avey, G. B., & Norman, S. M. (2007). Psychological capital: Developing positive psychological human resource practices. *The Academy of Management Review, 32*(1), 88–102.

Luthans, F., Avolio, B. J., & Avey, J. B. (2007). *Psychological capital questionnaire*. New York: Mind Garden, Inc.

Luthans, F., & Broad, J. D. (2022). Positive psychological capital to help combat the mental health fallout from the pandemic and VUCA environment. *Organizational Dynamics, 51*(2), 100817.

Luthans, F., & Youssef-Morgan, C. M. (2017). Psychological capital: An evidence-based positive approach. *Annual Review of Organizational Psychology and Organizational Behavior, 4*, 339–366.

Martins, R. M., & Gresse Von Wangenheim, C. (2023). Findings on teaching machine learning in high school: A ten-year systematic literature review. *Informatics in Education, 22*(3), 421–440.

McCanlies, E. C., Mnatsakanova, A., Andrew, M. E., Burchfiel, C. M., & Violanti, J. M. (2014). Positive psychological factors are associated with lower PTSD symptoms among police officers: Post Hurricane Katrina. *Stress and Health, 30*(5), 405–415. https://doi.org/10.1002/smi.2615.

Mukherjee, U., & Sharma, P. (2020). Hope at workplace: A review of literature. *International Journal of Psychosocial Rehabilitation, 24*(6), 557–5568.

National Alliance on Mental Illness. (2023). *Mental health conditions*. https://www.nami.org/Home.

National Institute of Justice. (2017, January). *Building and maintaining police officer resilience*.

Park, H., & Kim, J. Y. (2022). The predictive power of psychological capital dimensions for mental well-being among police officers: Implications for intervention development. *International Journal of Occupational Medicine and Environmental Health, 33*(1), 59–68.

Queiros, C., Passos, F., Bartolo, A., Marques, A. J., da Silva, C. F., & Pereira, A. (2020). Burnout and stress measurement in police officers: Literature review and a study with the operational police stress questionnaire. *Frontiers in Psychology, 11,* 587. https://doi.org/10.3389/fpsyg.2020.00587.

Satapathy, S. S. (2021). Social work research during COVID-19 pandemic: Understanding the issues and challenges of the corona warriors. *International Journal of Social and Development Concerns, 6.* Special Issue Social Work during COVID-19.

Sheridan, J., Xiao, W., & Chang, W. (2020). Mental health services and response in the context of COVID-19: A critical review. *International Journal of Mental Health Systems, 14*(1), 47.

Shirzad, H., Abbasi Farajzadeh, M., Hosseini Zijoud, S. R., & Farnoosh, G. (2020). The role of military and police forces in crisis management due to the COVID-19 outbreak in Iran and the world. *Journal of Police Medicine, 9*(2), 63–70.

Smith, J., & Jones, K. (2023). Gender disparities in psychological capital and mental well-being among police officers during the COVID-19 pandemic. *Journal of Police and Criminal Psychology, 38*(2), 123–135.

Stogner, J., Miller, B. L., & McLean, K. (2020). Police stress, mental health, and resiliency during the COVID-19 pandemic. *American Journal of Criminal Justice, 45*(4), 718–730. https://doi.org/10.1007/s12103-020-09548-y.Tehrani, N. (2022). The psychological impact of COVID-19 on police officers. *Criminal Justice and Policy Review, 33*(4), 506–525.

Telangana State Police. (n.d.). *Reference Handbook for Covid-19 Policing: Telangana State Police*. Indian Police Foundation. https://www.policefoundationindia.org/.

Tennant, R., Hiller, L., Fishwick, R., Platt, S., Joseph, S., Weich, S., & Stewart-Brown, S. (2007). The Warwick-Edinburgh mental well-being scale (WEMWBS): Development and UK validation. *Health and Quality of Life Outcomes, 5*(1), 1–13.

The Jed Foundation. (2023). *Promoting emotional well-being.*

Tiesman, H., Elkins, K., Brown, M., Marsh, S., & Carson, L. (2021). *Suicides among first responders: A call to action.* Centres for Disease Control and Prevention–NIOSH Science Blog.

Trujillo, S., Giraldo, L. S., López, J. D., Acosta, A., & Trujillo, N. (2021). Mental health outcomes in communities exposed to Armed Conflict Experiences. *BMC Psychology, 9*(1), 127. https://doi.10.1186/s40359-021-00626-2.

Walker, A., & Crawford, A. (2021). The impact of COVID-19 on police enforcement of public order offences. *British Journal of Criminology, 61*(4).

Wang, C., Horwitz, R. L., & Moskowitz, J. T. (2020). Frontline police officers and COVID-19: Potential occupational risks and mitigation strategies. *Journal of Police Science and Administration, 28*(2), 105–124.

World Health Organization (WHO). (2020a, March 11). *Mental health and COVID-19.*

World Health Organization (WHO). (2020b, March 11). *Novel Coronavirus (2019-nCoV) situation report – 40.* WHO.

World Health Organization (WHO). (2022). *The COVID-19 pandemic and mental health.* https://www.who.int/teams/mental-health-and-substance-use/mental-health-and-covid-19.

World Health Organization (WHO). (2023). *Mental health.* https://www.who.int/initiatives/who-special-initiative-for-mental-health.

8 Spiritual Tourism as a Panacea for Covid Burnout

A Review

Harshita Jha and Shaveta Sachdeva

Introduction

Burnout, a multifaceted phenomenon, has perhaps become synonymous with the COVID-19 pandemic that struck our lives in the past few years. In general, burnout can be understood as a state of being overextended and overwhelmed. It is described as a syndrome that includes the following three components: (1) emotional fatigue, (2) feelings of alienation or derealisation, and (3) a sense of inefficiency or lack of personal achievement (Restauri & Sheridan, 2020; Macaron et al., 2023). Peinado and Anderson (2020) describe burnout as part of everyday vocabulary, synonymous with stress. Although the researchers have made the above statement concerning social workers, it very well applies across different contexts and sections of populations. Previously, the concept of burnout was exclusively associated with the workplace or work-related stressors; however, today, the scenario is much more complex and far-reaching. Perhaps a more appropriate conceptualisation of burnout emerges from (Edú-valsania et al., 2022), who coined the term 'societal burnout' to describe the experience of the COVID-19 pandemic as an almost continuous assault on our bodies and minds. There was uncertainty, loss, fear, and even a sense of helplessness as we battled a grave societal threat.

COVID-19 will go down in history as a watershed event. It not only tested the limits of our physical healthcare infrastructure but also overstretched our mental, emotional, and psychological coping abilities. For instance, working from home became the norm, and the boundaries between personal and professional lives blurred (Sulaiman et al., 2022). Small and large organisations have adopted remote work in one swift, fast-paced transition. Even the places facilitating a sense of catharsis, community, and connectedness became out of reach for entire populations, with prominent religious festivals and pilgrimages banned (Ma et al., 2021). In a nutshell, our usual lifestyles, modes of communication and interaction, and daily routines all underwent vast amounts of change. This gap between unexpected changes (brought about by COVID-19) often went beyond our available coping abilities and resources, resulting in burnout-related symptoms (Figure 8.1).

This review examines the connection between spiritual health and COVID-19 burnout. It also discusses spiritual tourism as a novel strategy to treat burnout syndrome brought on by or made worse by the pandemic. Travel and tourism

DOI: 10.4324/9781003454984-9

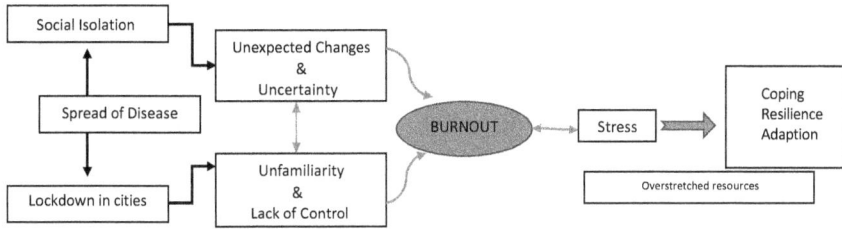

Figure 8.1 Burnout: Causes to Consequences.

can reshape individuals, encourage inward shifts, and mend broken personalities (Gezon, 2018). People care about their physical and mental well-being and strive to explore creative approaches to satisfy their requirements for happiness. Travel and tourism often become one such medium of self-discovery and fulfilment. After COVID-19, individuals will likely search for tourism options with specific therapeutic properties (Ma et al., 2021). Spiritual travel can promote healing and a sense of well-being. People become closer to nature and the natural world when they seek out isolation, retreat, and profound repair. These breathtaking scenes and natural settings can elicit strong emotional reactions and provide spiritual experiences. Thus, in the post-COVID-19 era, natural areas could be utilised by spiritual tourism (especially non-religious spiritual tourism) to offer a transformational solution. Nature-based and spiritual tourism can improve the lives of individuals (Gezon, 2018). Travelling to remote, natural areas away from the hustle and bustle of big cities is becoming increasingly popular. This development will benefit people's general and emotional well-being following COVID-19. Within this framework, the authors have suggested the following research questions:

Research Question 1: How can we understand burnout in light of COVID-19?

Research Question 2: How can spiritual health and burnout syndrome be related?

Research Question 3: What connections exist between spiritual tourism, burnout syndrome, and spiritual health?

Research Question 4: Can spiritual tourism be considered a COVID-19 mitigation strategy? What are the future research avenues for spiritual tourism post-COVID-19?

Methods

A literature review was conducted using several steps. A comprehensive search of several databases, including Google Scholar, PsycINFO, ProQuest, PubMed, and Dimensions AI, was performed (Table 8.1).

The following search strategy was used by the authors: (COVID-19 OR SARS-COV-2) AND (burnout), (COVID-19 OR SARS-COV-2) AND (spiritual health), (burnout) AND (spiritual health) AND COVID-19 OR SARS-COV-2,

Table 8.1 Search Strategy for Retrieving Data

Search	The Search Strategy Used in Database	Records Retrieved
1	COVID-19 OR SARS-COV-2 AND burnout	62,131
2	COVID-19 OR SARS-COV-2 AND spiritual health	77,446
3	COVID-19 OR SARS-COV-2 AND burnout AND spiritual health	1,180
4	COVID-19 OR SARS-COV-2 AND spiritual tourism	517

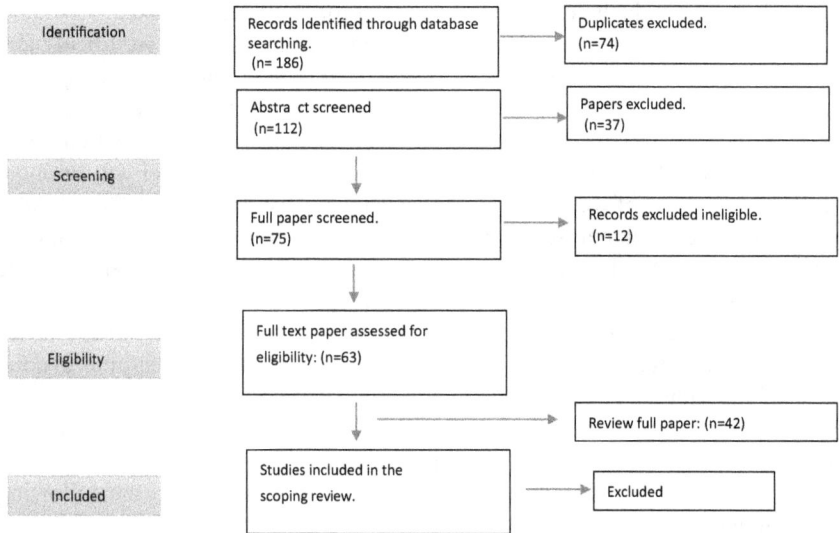

Figure 8.2 Workflow Chart.

(COVID-19 OR SARS-COV-2) AND (spiritual tourism) relevant to the chapter title, keywords, and abstract in the database. The authors used the Boolean operators "OR" to guarantee that the search returned results for all three queries and "AND" to guarantee that the search would contain at least one of the keywords "spiritual health", "spiritual tourism", and those related to the "pandemic".

The preliminary screening was done by authors independently, but the final selection of records was based on consensus. This agreement was based on inclusion and exclusion criteria and the authors' discretion. The inclusion criteria were (a) articles published from 2018 to 2023, (b) articles matching keywords in the title and abstracts, (c) peer-reviewed scientific articles, and (d) articles written in the English language. Any studies that did not include any of the above criteria were excluded. Finally, 75 scientific articles were identified as meeting the inclusion criteria mentioned above criteria. These were then put through further analysis (Figure 8.2 and Table 8.2).

Table 8.2 Result from the Search during 2018–2023 Using Dimensions AI, PsycINFO, PubMed

Author Name	Year	Title	Publication Resource	Citation
Abbas et al. (2021)	2022	Exploring the impact of COVID-19 on tourism: Transformational potential and implications for a sustainable recovery of the travel and leisure industry	Current Research in Behavioral Sciences, Elsevier	282
Ranjbari et al. (2021)	2021	Three pillars of sustainability in the wake of COVID-19: A systematic review and future research agenda for sustainable development	Journal of Cleaner Production, Elsevier	219
Pham et al. (2021)	2021	COVID-19 impacts of inbound tourism on Australian economy	Annals of Tourism Research, Elsevier	179
Yang et al. (2021)	2021	A review of early COVID-19 research in tourism: Launching the *Annals of Tourism Research*'s curated collection on coronavirus and tourism	Annals of Tourism Research, Elsevier	100
Mróz (2021)	2021	The impact of COVID-19 on pilgrimages and religious tourism in Europe during the first six months of the pandemic	Journal of Religion and Health, Springer	67
Wickramasinghe and Naranpanawa (2023)	2023	Tourism and COVID-19: An economy-wide assessment	Journal of Hospitality and Tourism Management, Elsevier	53
Christou et al. (2023)	2023	Spiritual tourism: Understandings, perspectives, discernment, and synthesis	Current Issue in Tourism, Taylor & Francis Online	43

Burnout Syndrome and COVID-19

The World Health Organisation's COVID-19 dashboard (2023) puts some glaring statistics before us. The severe acute respiratory syndrome coronavirus 2, abbreviated as (SARS-CoV-2) and related diseases (COVID-19) resulted in 774395,593 cases and over 7,023,271 deaths (as of 21 January 2024). These numbers are indicative of the countless households that were impacted on multiple levels - be it the loss of a loved one, financial strain, health comorbidities, social isolation, or loneliness, the list is never-ending. Given the severity and multidimensionality of the threats caused by COVID-19, one can expect negative emotional states to become more common shortly (Kumar & Nayar, 2020) cite the Indian Psychiatric Society's recent survey to highlight a substantial (almost 20%) rise in the number of mental health illnesses since the coronavirus outbreak. COVID-19 created an atmosphere of insecurity and scarcity. There were reports of household violence and hoarding of essential items such as masks and oxygen cylinders. Many people struggled for food, shelter, and their livelihoods. Globally, the pandemic was expected to increase the incidence of depression, anxiety disorders such as generalised anxiety disorders and obsessive-compulsive disorder, suicide rates, instances of self-harm, and alcohol addiction.

While the pandemic directly or indirectly impacted most individuals, most studies have explored burnout among frontline workers or health professionals. The category of healthcare workers is itself broad, often comprising physicians, nurses, emergency healthcare workers, intensive care unit specialists, and medical residents. Other communities, such as pharmacists, teachers, and entrepreneurs, have also been commonly studied. Even though burnout levels and stress symptoms were at an all-time high across different professions (Lind et al., 2023) due to the paucity of space and the scope of our work, the authors highlight the impact of COVID-19 on specific populations such as healthcare workers, teachers, and students. The list is not exhaustive. These studies, however, provide us with an overview of the complex and dynamic nature of COVID-19 and its linkages with burnout.

Originally, burnout was associated with jobs characterised by high-stress levels. During the pandemic, healthcare jobs became one of the most stressful professions as they involved regular contact with infected patients, long hours of duty, excessive workload, arduous protection gear, and concerns regarding their health and the well-being of their family members (Ferry et al., 2021).

Studies have shown that burnout levels were higher among medical staff dealing with critically ill patients. A larger proportion of nurses experienced burnout than physicians.

Additionally, medical staff originally posted in the emergency departments or urgent care centres were more likely to have moderate-to-severe burnout levels than staff members who were deployed (Chor et al., 2021).

Similarly, Matsuo et al. (2020) found the prevalence of psychological strain and burnout among laboratory medical technologists, radiological technologists, and pharmacists working with COVID-19 patients in Japan. According to Ghahramani et al.'s systematic review and meta-analytic study (2021), emotional exhaustion was more prevalent in non-frontline workers, while frontline workers had higher depersonalisation and lack of personal achievement prevalence. Their findings are interesting as they indicate that irrespective of whether or not health professionals dealt with COVID-19 patients, a certain level of burnout was experienced across hospital staff. Apart from being physically strenuous, COVID-19 generally resulted in increased levels of burnout, anxiety, and depression among healthcare workers, especially the ones working with infected patients. Predictably, previous pandemic encounters (involving similar contagion trajectories) suggest that healthcare workers are prone to developing symptoms of anxiety, post-traumatic stress disorder, insomnia, depression, and substance use disorders (Müller et al., 2023). These mental health challenges are reported across different populations and geographies. For instance, among Chinese healthcare workers, nurses, women, and frontline healthcare workers exposed to COVID-19 experienced the highest risk of developing the most unfavourable mental health outcomes, including anxiety, depression, distress and insomnia (Lai et al., 2020). However, some studies have also reported that physicians actively engaged in the battle against COVID-19 had lower levels of burnout and high satisfaction with work, along with a greater sense of personal accomplishment, as they perceived their work as meaningful and they could see immediate outcomes for their effort (Dinibutun, 2020).

The pandemic also resulted in the overhaul of school and higher education systems. The education sector encountered an overwhelming set of challenges due to mobility restrictions and social distancing norms in place. Teachers are, of course, the backbone of any educational setting. Therefore, they were expected to quickly adapt to their roles as educators, new instructional approaches, and hybrid classroom settings. Pressley (2021) thinks that teachers experienced numerous stressors during COVID-19 that directly affected their levels of stress and anxiety. The implications of high burnout levels are far and wide, as many studies have shown that teachers with high burnout have more disagreements with their students, there is less satisfaction in their student-pupil relationships, and their students perform poorly academically. Teachers exhibiting burnout symptoms were likely to demonstrate lesser engagement with students, restricted social interaction in class, reduced involvement in teaching/curriculum planning, and decreased motivation. They may also tend to make more negative evaluations of their students than someone who is not experiencing burnout (Sokal et al., 2021), adversely affecting student learning outcomes and the environment (Tomaszek & Muchacka-Cymerman, 2022). The study highlighted the fact that during the COVID-19 epidemic, young people faced additional risks that have had an impact on their entire functioning and worldview. It appears that the COVID-19 pandemic has exacerbated the existing symptoms of anxiety and burnout, thus further adding to their trauma.

From the findings mentioned above, it was inferred that burnout's physical and psychosocial impacts have received considerable attention. The pandemic experience, however, has taught us that our experience of 'health and well-being' can go beyond these aspects. At a time when death and suffering had become the norm, people began to delve into more profound spiritual questions that attempt to understand the mysteries of our existence and our connection to a higher power. The following section explores the relationship between COVID-19 and spiritual health.

COVID-19 and Spiritual Health: Exploring Linkages

The World Health Organisation defines health as a "state of complete physical, mental and social wellbeing and not merely the absence of disease or infirmity." The human experience also goes beyond the physical, mental, and social aspects to include those dimensions of well-being that are intangible, meta-physical, or existential yet can be described as one of the critical aspects of health and wellbeing. In other words, spiritual health can be said to encompass those aspects of health that are not physical, psychological, or social. Ghaderi et al. (2018) have proposed three aspects of spiritual health: the religious component, the individualistic component or connection with oneself, and the material world-oriented or the connection with others/natural world. Further, they have elaborated on the components of spiritual health reflected within four domains of the connection between God (transcendent reality) and humans, connection with one's selves, others, and nature. In general, spiritual needs encompass those aspects of our lives wherein we seek connection and belongingness to the universe or larger entity; it is associated with feelings of peace and a life of meaning and value.

The pandemic caused profound disruption, confusion, and existential anxiety in most people. It pushed those with spiritual anguish into periods of doubt and questioning, wherein they tried to understand the nature of suffering and their relationship with it (Coppola et al., 2021). The relationship between COVID-19 and spiritual health is multifaceted. On the one hand, the stress and uncertainty brought about by the pandemic led individuals to turn to their spiritual beliefs and practices as a source of comfort and guidance (Samełko et al., 2023). Engaging in spiritual activities, such as meditation, prayer, or attending virtual religious congregations or services, can provide comfort and a sense of connection to something greater than oneself.

Additionally, spiritual health can contribute to individuals' well-being during the pandemic by fostering resilience and providing hope and purpose. On the other hand, COVID-19 has also disrupted traditional forms of religious worship and community gatherings, creating challenges for individuals to practice their spirituality in the same ways they did before. It led to the emergence of new and innovative approaches to spiritual practice, such as virtual religious services and online meditation groups. These adaptations have allowed individuals to maintain their spiritual health and connection, albeit in different ways.

Exploring the linkages between COVID-19 and spiritual health can provide insights into how individuals find meaning, cope with stress, and maintain resilience during these challenging times. This can help inform strategies for promoting holistic well-being and supporting individuals in navigating the emotional and psychological impacts of the pandemic. By investigating COVID-19's impact on individuals' spirituality and religious practices, we can better understand how this global crisis has influenced their perceptions, beliefs, and behaviours. One means of promoting spiritual health and pursuing spiritual needs is engaging in spiritual tourism. The following section illuminates the concept of spiritual tourism and its motives.

Understanding Spiritual Tourism and Its Motives

We know that travel and holidays are frequently seen as ways to decompress and revitalise the monotonous daily grind. They become a source of traveller's happy emotional states. Understanding the phenomenon of spiritual tourism and its goals is crucial for appreciating how religious travel is changing and how it affects travellers looking for distinctive experiences, cultural enrichment, and individual development (Halim et al., 2021). A specific travel category connected to a person's religious beliefs is known as spiritual tourism. Tourists and pilgrims have traditionally been seen as two distinct groups in the field of tourism studies due to their different motivations for travel and destination preferences.

For example, pilgrims are drawn to holy places for spiritual and religious reasons, whereas tourists travel for hedonistic pleasures and secular interests (Yousaf, 2021). However, modern travel and tourism literature does not divide tourists into binary categories of pilgrims and tourists; this implies that the reasons for travelling may not define the nature of a tourist, as sometimes people travel for reasons that are mixed and complex. Travel done for religious purposes can be considered a type of special interest tourism.

Spiritual tourism as a term is often used interchangeably with religious tourism. Since ancient times, people have travelled across geographies for religion-related purposes, making religiously motivated travel one of the oldest motives behind cross-border mobility (Mróz, 2021). However, while religious tourism is usually centred around an object of devotion (deity/symbol/relic/sacred place) that is valued in a particular religion, spiritual tourism is undertaken with the primary objective of the inner journey of self-exploration and an effort to find meaning and purpose in existence. It may or may not involve any religious object or ritual. In this context, religious tourism can also be included as part of spiritual tourism. Today, it has become crucial to look at the drivers of spiritual tourism as it becomes increasingly evident that pilgrimages to holy places are not just driven by religious fervour. Fulfilment of one's spiritual needs and the charged other-worldly atmosphere of religious places have emerged as primary priority motives behind spiritual travel (Garg et al., 2021). However, travelling to holy locations is also motivated by other factors, like enjoying the flora, fauna, and landscape, achieving educational/information-based or socio-cultural goals, unwinding, engaging in self-care and rejuvenation, and spending time in and around nature (Garg et al., 2021), thus expanding the ambit of spiritual tourism.

Results

The current literature review emphasised the significance of spiritual health in day-to-day tourist activities during the COVID-19 pandemic. Tourism is one of the most affected industries by the pandemic, with a staggering 80% drop in international arrivals from January 2020 to January 2021 (UNWTO World Tourism Barometer and Statistical Annex, March 2021, 2021). For many years, the older generation in India has been interested in spiritual travel. This has changed in the last year and a half, i.e., around 2023–2022, with new-age, younger travellers seeking to detach from regular life. Spiritual retreats that offer a combination of religious and off-the-grid locations provide a perfect atmosphere for detoxifying the soul and mind. The spiritual journey appears to begin in a world of uncertainty, infinite distractions, and terrible anguish. It seems that COVID-19

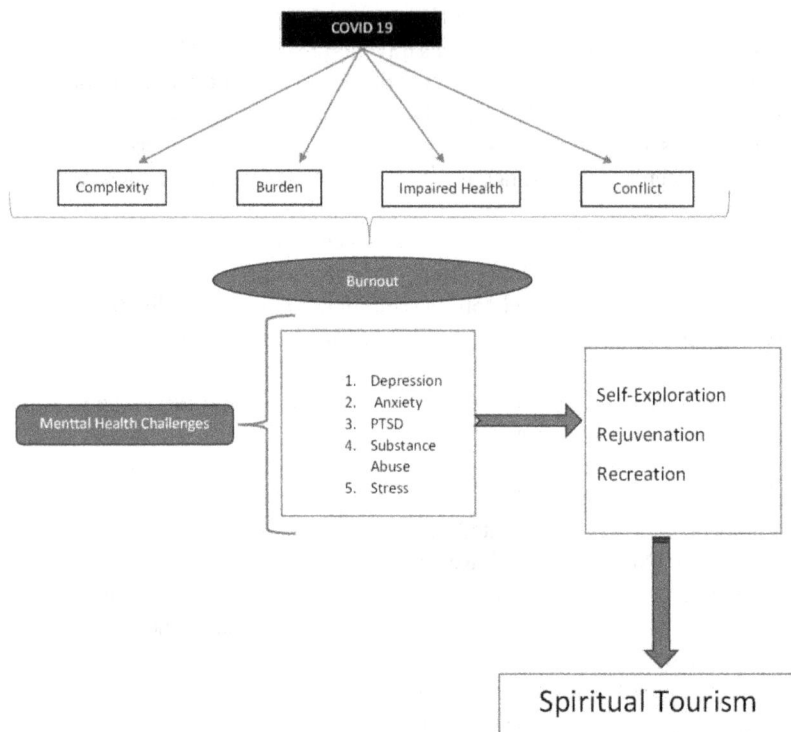

Figure 8.3 Factors Associated with COVID-19 Burnout and Their Links to Spiritual Tourism.

and its disruption offered a fertile ground for individuals to reconnect with their spiritual health.

With the pandemic receding, both domestic and international destinations have reopened for tourists, and as per the latest trends, spiritual tourism is the next big trend in 2023. Spiritual tourism is an active pursuit of spirituality through travel and tourism-related activities. Spiritual tourism has also increasingly captured the interest of academicians, with an increase in the number of studies around the same themes. More and more researchers are trying to understand human being's quest towards self-knowledge and inquiry through spiritual or religious travel (Christou et al., 2023). Further, some studies highlighted that in COVID-19, perhaps one of the most valuable resources tourists possess is their faith, trust, and spirituality. Based on the literature review, the following framework of spiritual tourism to cope with COVID-19 burnout has been established (Figure 8.3):

Lockdowns imposed during COVID-19 meant restricted mobility. As time and resources rapidly depleted for the tourists, the travel goals, even to religious/spiritual sites, remained unfulfilled (Abbas et al., 2021). Additionally, it was thought that the fear engendered by the pandemic depletes people's mental capacities, impairing their capacity for everyday tasks and their standard of living (Pocinho et al., 2022).

People were confined to one location during the COVID-19 pandemic, which led to a large number of psychological and mental issues. Duarte (2020) found that higher levels of life satisfaction were significantly associated with lower levels of all dimensions of burnout. This implies that since COVID-19 severely hampered the quality of life for most people, burnout levels were also on the rise for different populations during the pandemic.

Eventually, as people ventured outside their houses and resumed travel, they sought to combine pleasure and enjoyment with deeper spiritual needs. In a way, spiritual tourism addressed the boredom and monotony that gripped most of us as we were imprisoned by our daily routines and multiple social restrictions during lockdown. Improved acceptance and contentment were some of the additional benefits that could be experienced through spiritual tourism. The following section highlights the potential drivers of spiritual tourism and its larger role in well-being and economy.

Discussion

The goal of the current study was to comprehend burnout syndrome in the context of COVID-19. It also explored the relationship between burnout syndrome and spiritual well-being. The authors also examined any possible connections between burnout syndrome, spiritual wellness, and spiritual tourism. Spiritual tourism was studied as a unique approach to mitigate the effects of COVID-19. Future directions for spiritual tourism were also considered.

It is important to note that travel for spiritual purposes not only refreshes and renews our sense of marvel, but it is also fundamentally linked to the concept of self-care and a deeper connection to the planet, with other people, and even with oneself. The desire and search for happiness and fulfilment in society are stronger than ever, and the longing to explore the spiritual world has gathered a new momentum.

The motivation behind spiritual tourism can vary greatly depending on the individuals and their beliefs. Earlier studies have shown the spiritual components of visiting religious sites and the drivers behind them. These studies have demonstrated, for instance, that Muslims may be inspired to travel to Umrah to partake in religious rituals and adopt lifestyles that are consistent with their spiritual beliefs, the Hindus may visit temples or sites of historical importance or the ones mentioned as significant by their ancient scriptures and, likewise, the Buddhists are also known to travel to holy sites linked to Buddha's relics and life-journey. In tourism, studies examining motivations seek to explore the justification for conducting travel adventures and to outline travel behaviour. The allocentric-psychometric model of Plog, the push-pull factor framework of Dann, the escape-seeking model by Ross & Iso-Ahola, and the travel career ladder model by Pearce and Lee (Garg et al., 2021) are just a few of the models and theories on which several studies on the motivations of tourists are based. Motives behind spiritual tourism can include seeking spiritual enlightenment, experiencing sacred or holy places, connecting with one's inner self, engaging in religious rituals or practices, seeking personal growth and transformation, or simply finding peace and tranquillity, the spiritual tourism also crosses religious barriers, making it a varied and inclusive kind of travel that is unrestricted by a person's particular

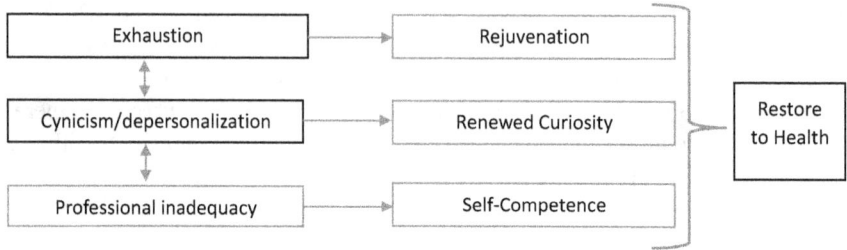

Figure 8.4 Spiritual Tourism Addressing COVID-19 Burnout.

religion, belief system, location, or nation. The motives were varied, but overall, they can facilitate coping with symptoms of burnout in tourists who undertake this journey. The following framework mentions the primary motivating factors that can address COVID-19 burnout (Figure 8.4):

At a time when the tourism industry at large continues to traverse its recovery journey, designing innovative tourism activities in alignment with the diverse needs of individuals and groups can offer the much-needed boost to the tourist sector and overall economy (Abbas et al., 2021). To ensure a steady recovery of the tourism industry, it is also essential to forecast tourism demand. Considering that tourism is a significant driver of growth across countries and regions (Pham et al., 2021), understanding the needs and expectations of tourists can enable better planning and channelling of resources when it comes to developing specific sites for tourist activities (Hu et al., 2021; Yang et al., 2021). As the world opens up, people are increasingly preparing to engage in wellness tourism activities in the post-pandemic period as they begin to research health and wellness options online. Focus on travel that centres around building well-being and resilience, ensuring safety and access to relatively secluded and under-crowded places, is touted as the next big trend likely to drive tourist behaviour in upcoming years (Pocinho et al., 2022). There is an exponential increase in the realisation that engaging in spiritual tourism activities is crucial for restoring physical and mental health. People are more health-conscious than before, making spiritual and wellness retreats one of the most coveted vacation choices. It is understood to rejuvenate the visitors via healthy food, maintaining connections with oneself and the environment, and offering an all-encompassing genuine experience.

In this study, with tourism directed at spiritual activities, researchers intended to gain a deeper understanding of the many factors that influence people's desire to engage in spiritual tourism, including their appreciation of nature, their desire to further their education or experience another culture, their need for relaxation and self-care, and their desire to spend time in nature.

Limitations of the Study and Future Directions

The authors primarily covered literature about the larger themes around COVID-19, burnout and tourism, and not spiritual tourism in particular. One of the reasons for this is the need for studies that have directly explored the concept of spiritual tourism, especially as a coping strategy for dealing with burnout symptoms. The study, however, has attempted to establish spiritual tourism as one of the alternative strategies to help individuals and groups overcome post-pandemic fatigue. It is suggested that future studies in this area explore the impact of spiritual tourism on tourists' mental, psychological, and emotional well-being, tourist behaviour, and stress and burnout-related symptoms. Researchers interested in this area can also explore spiritual tourism's economic and financial contribution or implication, specifically concerning the tourism industry and the larger economy.

While COVID-19 may have become the lens through which a lot of pre–post-pandemic comparisons are being conducted using a multitude of variables, as academicians and researchers, it is also equally important to realise that COVID-19 (however significant) is but a transitory wave in an ever-changing world (Yang et al., 2021). This implies immense scope exists to understand the interlinkages between spiritual health, burnout and spiritual tourism beyond the pandemic.

Conclusion

The authors have attempted to introduce spiritual tourism as one of the coping strategies to address COVID-19 burnout and its after-effects or consequences. The present work offers an unexplored dimension of healing and rejuvenation embedded in linkages between burnout, spiritual health, and spiritual tourism. Spiritual assistance can help individuals and families cope with COVID-19-led psychological and physical illnesses. Numerous research studies have identified spiritual practices as effective coping strategies for handling traumatic and life-altering experiences (Roman et al., 2020). The authors believe in the unique potential of using spiritual tourism as a coping strategy or therapeutic element to deal with COVID-19 burnout and its effects. There is scope for studying spiritual tourism as a variable concerning health, burnout, stress, and well-being. According to studies on the advantages of spiritual coping, it is conceivable that including spiritual tourism during this challenging moment might give people a special chance for recovery, renewal, and the restoration of mental well-being.

Furthermore, there are several types of studies addressing the burnout syndrome that occurred during the COVID-19 pandemic, indicating that healthcare professionals and teachers were particularly vulnerable due to the demanding nature of their profession and work environment, including other professions, employed/unemployed categories to explore the level and severity of burnout in different sections of society. COVID-19 burnout should be studied across different demographics and cultures to understand each group's unique challenges and risk factors. In other words, by studying burnout syndrome across different professions, populations, and cultures during the COVID-19 pandemic, researchers can better understand the unique challenges and factors contributing to burnout in various contexts (Pujiyanto et al., 2022). This understanding can inform the development and implementation of relevant support systems and targeted interventions to allay burnout and promote overall well-being.

Tourism in itself may not be a one-stop solution to address something as complex as burnout. However, there is reasonable evidence in the literature that it can contribute as one of the alternate strategies to reduce burnout levels and promote health and well-being for a population struggling with the after-effects of the pandemic.

Acknowledgements

The authors would like to express their heartfelt gratitude to the academic advisors and anonymous peer reviewers who have dedicated their valuable time and expertise to provide constructive feedback on this chapter. Their insightful comments have greatly contributed to the quality of this study.

References

Abbas, J., Mubeen, R., Iorember, P. T., Raza, S., & Mamirkulova, G. (2021). Exploring the impact of COVID-19 on tourism: transformational potential and implications for a sustainable recovery of the travel and leisure industry. *Current Research in Behavioral Sciences, 2*. https://doi.org/10.1016/j.crbeha.2021.100033

Chor, W. P. D., Ng, W. M., Cheng, L., Situ, W., Chong, J. W., Ng, L. Y. A., et al. (2021). Burnout amongst emergency healthcare workers during the COVID-19 pandemic: A multi-center study. *American Journal of Emergency Medicine, 46*, 700–702. https://doi.org/10.1016/j.ajem.2020.10.040

Christou, P. A., Pericleous, K., & Singleton, A. (2023). Spiritual tourism: Understandings, perspectives, discernment, and synthesis. *Current Issues in Tourism, 26*(20), 3288–3305. https://doi.org/10.1080/13683500.2023.2183819

Coppola, I., Rania, N., Parisi, R., & Lagomarsino, F. (2021). Spiritual well-being and mental health during the COVID-19 pandemic in Italy. *Frontiers in Psychiatry, 12*. https://doi.org/10.3389/FPSYT.2021.626944

Dinibutun, S. R. (2020). Factors associated with burnout among physicians: An evaluation during a period of COVID-19 pandemic. *Journal of Healthcare Leadership, 12*, 85. https://doi.org/10.2147/JHL.S270440

Duarte, I., Alves, A., Coelho, A., Ferreira, A., Cabral, B., Silva, B., Peralta, J., Silva, J., Domingues, P., Nunes, P., Serrão, C., & Santos, C. (2022). The mediating role of resilience and life satisfaction in the relationship between stress and burnout in medical students during the COVID-19 pandemic. *International Journal of Environmental Research and Public Health, 19*(5), 2822. https://doi.org/10.3390/ijerph19052822

Edú-valsania, S., Laguía, A., & Moriano, J. A. (2022). Burnout: A review of theory and measurement. *International Journal of Environmental Research and Public Health, 19*(3). https://doi.org/10.3390/IJERPH19031780

Ferry, A. V., Wereski, R., Strachan, F. E., & Mills, N. L. (2021). Predictors of UK healthcare worker burnout during the COVID-19 pandemic. *QJM, 114*(6), 374–380. https://doi.org/10.1093/qjmed/hcab065

Garg, A., Misra, P., Gupta, S., Goel, P., & Saleem, M. (2021). Prioritising motivators influencing intentions to visit spiritual destinations in India: An application of analytical hierarchical process (AHP) approach. *Journal of Tourism Futures*, 1–16. https://doi.org/10.1108/JTF-09-2021-0214

Gezon, L. L. (2018). Global scouts: youth engagement with spirituality and wellness through travel, Lake Atitlán, Guatemala. *Journal of Tourism and Cultural Change, 16*(4), 365–378. https://doi.org/10.1080/14766825.2017.1310217

Ghaderi, A., Tabatabaei, S. M., Nedjat, S., Javadi, M., & Larijani, B. (2018). Explanatory definition of the concept of spiritual health: A qualitative study in Iran. *Journal of Medical Ethics and History of Medicine, 11*(3).

Ghahramani, S., Lankarani, K. B., Yousefi, M., Heydari, K., Shahabi, S., & Azmand, S. (2021). A systematic review and meta-analysis of burnout among healthcare workers during COVID-19. *Frontiers in Psychiatry, 12*, 758849. https://doi.org/10.3389/fpsyt.2021.758849

Halim, M. S. A., Tatoglu, E., & Hanefar, S. B. M. (2021). A review of spiritual tourism: A conceptual model for future research. *Tourism and Hospitality Management, 27*(1), 119–141. https://doi.org/10.20867/thm.27.1.8

Hu, F., Teichert, T., Deng, S., Liu, Y., & Zhou, G. (2021). Dealing with pandemics: An investigation of the effects of COVID-19 on customers' evaluations of hospitality services. *Tourism Management, 85*. https://doi.org/10.1016/j.tourman.2021.104320

Kumar, A., & Nayar, K. R. (2020). COVID-19 and its mental health consequences. *Journal of Mental Health, 30*(1), 1–2. https://doi.org/10.1080/09638237.2020.1757052

Lai, J., Ma, S., Wang, Y., Cai, Z., Hu, J., Wei, N., et al. (2020). Factors associated with mental health outcomes among health care workers exposed to coronavirus disease 2019. *JAMA Network Open, 3*(3). https://doi.org/10.1001/JAMANETWORKOPEN.2020.3976

Lind, L. M., Ward, R. N., Rose, S. G., & Brown, L. M. (2023). The impact of the COVID-19 pandemic on psychological service provision, mental health practitioners, and patients in long-term care settings: Results from a rapid response survey. *Professional Psychology: Research and Practice, 54*(1), 93–102. https://doi.org/10.1037/pro0000486

Ma, S., Zhao, X., Gong, Y., & Wengel, Y. (2021). Proposing "healing tourism" as a post-COVID-19 tourism product. *Anatolia, 32*(1), 136–139. https://doi.org/10.1080/13032917.2020.1808490

Macaron, M. M., Segun-Omosehin, O. A., Matar, R. H., Beran, A., Nakanishi, H., Than, C. A., & Abulseoud, O. A. (2023). A systematic review and meta-analysis on burnout in physicians during the COVID-19 pandemic: A hidden healthcare crisis. *Frontiers in Psychiatry, 13*(January). https://doi.org/10.3389/fpsyt.2022.1071397

Matsuo, T., Kobayashi, D., Taki, F., Sakamoto, F., Uehara, Y., Mori, N., & Fukui, T. (2020). Prevalence of health care worker burnout during the coronavirus disease 2019 (COVID-19) pandemic in Japan. *JAMA Network Open, 3*(8), e2017271–e2017271. https://doi.org/10.1001/JAMANETWORKOPEN.2020.17271

Mróz, F. (2021). The impact of COVID-19 on pilgrimages and religious tourism in Europe during the first six months of the pandemic. *Journal of Religion and Health, 60*(2), 625–645. https://doi.org/10.1007/S10943-021-01201-0/FIGURES/7

Müller, M. M., Baillès, E., Blanch, J., Torres, X., Rousaud, A., Cañizares, S., et al. (2023). Burnout among hospital staff during the COVID-19 pandemic: Longitudinal results from the international Cope-Corona survey study. *Journal of Psychosomatic Research, 164*(August 2022). https://doi.org/10.1016/j.jpsychores.2022.111102

Peinado, M., & Anderson, K. N. (2020). Reducing social worker burnout during COVID-19. *International Social Work, 63*(6), 757–760. https://doi.org/10.1177/0020872820962196

Pham, T. D., Dwyer, L., Su, J. J., & Ngo, T. (2021). COVID-19 impacts of inbound tourism on Australian economy. *Annals of Tourism Research, 88*, 103179. https://doi.org/10.1016/j.annals.2021.103179

Pocinho, M., Garcês, S., & de Jesus, S. N. (2022). Wellbeing and resilience in tourism: A systematic literature review during COVID-19. *Frontiers in Psychology, 12.* Frontiers Media S.A. https://doi.org/10.3389/fpsyg.2021.748947

Pressley, T. (2021). Factors contributing to teacher burnout during COVID-19. *Educational Researcher, 50*(5), 325–327. https://doi.org/10.3102/0013189X211004138

Pujiyanto, T. I., Mendrofa, F. A. M. & Hani, U. (2022). Burnout among nurses working in COVID-19 pandemic. *International Journal of Public Health Science, 11*(1), 113–120. https://doi.org/10.11591/ijphs.v11i1.21267

Ranjbari, M., Shams Esfandabadi, Z., Zanetti, M. C., Scagnelli, S. D., Siebers, P. O., Aghbashlo, M., et al. (2021). Three pillars of sustainability in the wake of COVID-19: A systematic review and future research agenda for sustainable development. *Journal of Cleaner Production, 297*, 126660. https://doi.org/10.1016/j.jclepro.2021.126660

Restauri, N., & Sheridan, A. D. (2020). Burnout and posttraumatic stress disorder in the coronavirus disease 2019 (COVID-19) pandemic: Intersection, impact, and interventions. *Journal of the American College of Radiology, 17*(7), 921–926. https://doi.org/10.1016/j.jacr.2020.05.021

Roman, N. V., Mthembu, T. G., & Hoosen, M. (2020). Spiritual care - 'A deeper immunity' - A response to Covid-19 pandemic. *African Journal of Primary Health Care & Family Medicine, 12*(1), e1–e3. https://doi.org/10.4102/phcfm.v12i1.2456

Samełko, A., Woycikiewicz, M. D. B., & Kenioua, M. (2023). Physical activity and selected psychological constructs of intercultural students in the field of physical education during the Covid-19 pandemic. *Physical Culture and Sport, Studies and Research, 98*(1), 1–12. https://doi.org/10.2478/pcssr-2023-0001

Sokal, L., Trudel, L. E., & Babb, J. (2021). I've had it! Factors associated with burnout and low organizational commitment in Canadian teachers during the second wave of the COVID-19 pandemic. *International Journal of Educational Research Open, 2*(December 2020), 100023. https://doi.org/10.1016/j.ijedro.2020.100023

Sulaiman, R., Mohammed Zabidi, M., Hj. Basri, F., Mohd Marzuki, Z., Mohd Zin, M. Z., & Ozata, S. (2022). Work burnout and spiritual well-being during Covid-19 pandemic amongst staff in two Malaysian public universities. *International Journal of Academic Research in Business and Social Sciences, 12*(5), 1555–1569. https://doi.org/10.6007/ijarbss/v12-i5/13247

Tomaszek, K., & Muchacka-Cymerman, A. (2022). Student burnout and PTSD symptoms: The role of existential anxiety and academic fears on students during the COVID-19 pandemic. *Depression Research and Treatment, 2022.* https://doi.org/10.1155/2022/6979310

UNWTO World Tourism Barometer and Statistical Annex, March 2021. (2021). *UNWTO World Tourism Barometer, 19*(2), 1–32. https://doi.org/10.18111/WTOBARO METERENG.2021.19.1.2

Wickramasinghe, K., & Naranpanawa, A. (2023). Tourism and COVID-19: An economy-wide assessment. *Journal of Hospitality and Tourism Management, 55*, 131–138. https://doi.org/10.1016/J.JHTM.2023.03.013

Yang, Y., Zhang, C. X., & Rickly, J. M. (2021). A review of early COVID-19 research in tourism: Launching the Annals of Tourism Research's Curated Collection on coronavirus and tourism. *Annals of Tourism Research, 91*, 103313. https://doi.org/10.1016/j.annals.2021.103313

Yousaf, S. (2021). Travel burnout: Exploring the return journeys of pilgrim-tourists amidst the COVID-19 pandemic. *Tourism Management, 84*(January), 104285. https://doi.org/10.1016/j.tourman.2021.104285

9 Rajyoga Meditation as an Intervention Technique for Managing Negative Affect Post-COVID-19

Pavitra Singh and Pradeep Kumar

Introduction

The COVID-19 pandemic had widespread effects across the globe, affecting almost all nations and territories; it was more than a health crisis. People have been affected mentally, socially, economically, and physically to a great extent. The lockdown restrictions in response to the contagious virus impacted everyone's routine activities, and a wave of fear was seen across the globe (Pulla, 2020). As per the scientific report by the World Health Organisation (WHO), there was a 25% increase in the worldwide incidence of anxiety and depression during the first year of the COVID-19-led pandemic (WHO, 2022). Mental health holds incredible importance amid the COVID-19 pandemic. Blending spiritual awareness and emotional intelligence (Mayer, 2000) was desired to manage well-being during the pandemic. Meditation plays a significant role in developing an emotional immune system that can protect against internal crises and maintain unperturbed well-being. With the practice of yogic meditation, respiration exhibits synchronisation (Braboszcz et al., 2010), and the cardiac rhythm reverts to its standard range (Levine et al., 2017), contributing to the regulation of hypertension and a reduction in the psychosomatic manifestations of diseases, as well as the necessary pharmacological dosage (Satsangi & Brugnoli, 2018; Shanker et al., 2018).

Moreover, it was also found that there is a decrease in the concentration of lactic acid in the bloodstream, systolic blood pressure gravitates towards a normal range, immunological defences are enhanced, and muscular tension is alleviated (Patel, 1996). Rajyoga is concentrative meditation designed to discipline lifestyle, mind, and body (Rao, 2012). Eight steps are popularly known as the Eight-Limbed Model/Eight-Fold Path of Yoga. The process of reaching the highest state of consciousness is by following the eight steps in meditative form; they are as follows: yamas, niyama (moral-cum-ethical principles), asana and pranayama (purifying the body and breath), pratyahara (being detached from senses), dharana dhyana and samadhi (meditative state). Sage 'Patanjali' is considered the father of Yogic Meditation. He was the first to systematically codify aphorisms (sutras) on yoga in eight consecutive steps called Ashtanga Yoga/Rajyoga (Prabhavananda & Isherwood, 1948). It is the oldest yoga system with a systematic approach to controlling the fluctuations of the mind. In the 19th century, Swami Vivekananda interpreted Patanjali's Yoga

DOI: 10.4324/9781003454984-10

Sutras in his book Raja Yoga (Yogeshwar, 1994), which gave yoga a modern name. However, the ultimate goal of yoga philosophy goes beyond physical and emotional well-being and advances toward the realm of spiritual realisation. Rajyoga provides a comprehensive compendium of psychological concepts and mind-body techniques to help overcome sadness, suffering, and pain, especially during the COVID-19 pandemic (Bhide et al., 2022; Padhan, 2022). Psychological problems like anxiety, depression, and fear can be reduced by the practice of Rajyoga meditation (Araujo et al., 2021; Arora & Girgila, 2014; Varambally & Gangadhar, 2012). Further, it has been discovered that Rajyoga meditation induces neural plasticity in the cerebral cortex, analogous to skill acquisition (Lazar et al., 2005). It also modulates the cortisol concentration in patients subjected to surgical procedures (Kiran et al., 2017). Rajyoga meditation has been shown to enhance one's sense of well-being (Chouhan & Singh, 2021; Singh et al., 2021; Nair et al., 2018). In addition, it has been observed that Rajyoga meditation can be effective in managing stress and anxiety, particularly during the COVID-19 pandemic (Madhu et al., 2022; Jain, 2020). Furthermore, listening to spiritual music has been found to induce a sense of tranquillity and peace due to its uplifting lyrics, as Sekhsaria (2020) noted.

Numerous researchers have suggested the potential of developing a therapy rooted in Patanjali's Yoga Sutra as a solution for mental health disorders (Latha, 2014; Chowdhary & Gopinath, 2013; Balodhi & Chowdhary, 1986). Therefore, the present study attempts to develop an intervention by incorporating eight limbs into a meditative form, as meditation plays a vital role in internalising the teaching of Yoga Sutra into daily life. This intervention is based on Patanjali's Eight-Limbed Model, a comprehensive meditation manual that guides a balanced and ethical life (Pizer, 2023). The previous findings suggest that consistent engagement in meditation, asana, and pranayama can effectively mitigate negative emotions, such as stress, anxiety, depression, and fear (Madhu et al., 2022; Varambally & Gangadhar, 2012; Lemay et al., 2019; Patel, 1996). Furthermore, it has been found that maintaining a meditation practice for at least 30 days can improve mental health and decrease psychological distress and anxiety (Madhu et al., 2022; Jain, 2020).

Objective: To assess the effectiveness of Rajyoga Meditation Intervention on Negative Affect, based on Patanjali's Yoga Sutra.

H_1: There would be a decrease in Negative Affect after the Rajyoga Meditation Intervention.

Method

Design: The study used a quasi-experimental, single-group (within-group) pre–post-test design. The sampling technique was convenient sampling.

Participants: Eighty-seven participants from Vipul World Society Gurugram, Haryana (India) took part in the study, out of which 74 (62 females and 12 males) continued with sessions over eight weeks. The intervention took place in Vipul World Hall. Participants who were approachable and committed to being consistent for eight weeks were recruited. The age range was 26–67 (average age 48.4 years).

Given pre–post-testing of negative affect, the self-reported instrument Eight State Questionnaire (8SQ) by Curran and Cattell (1976) was administered for data collection. It consists of 96 items measuring eight mood states: Stress, Anxiety, Depression, Fatigue, Regression, Guilt, Arousal, and Extraversion. This assessment tool does not provide a cumulative score for negative affect. Instead, it evaluates six types of negative affect, each representing a different facet of this complex psychological construct. In addition to these six types of negative affect, the assessment also measures two other mood states: arousal and extraversion. These are not negative affect, but they are included in the assessment to provide a more comprehensive picture of the individual's emotional state.

Interestingly, the scores for these two mood states are inversely related. The assessment is designed to apply to a wide age range. It is suitable for adults and adolescents 16 years or older, making it a versatile tool for psychological evaluation. The 8SQ measurement tool is notably sensitive to changes in the mood-related responses of participants. As a result, it has been considered crucial to control external elements that could affect mood carefully. Controlling was taken care of by taking timely feedback from participants to confirm that the observed alterations in the participants' mood states were genuinely due to the intervention rather than unrelated factors like personal reasons.

Inclusion–exclusion criteria: Participants who self-reported as not suffering from physical/mental illness and not undergoing any treatment were included. Participants who joined any other meditation program were excluded from the sample.

Procedure: The Rajyoga meditation intervention spanned eight weeks, each day consisting of a 45-minute (offline) session post-COVID-19. These sessions were structured to include an initial 15 minutes for cognitive training, followed by 20 minutes dedicated to meditation practice, and concluding with a 10-minute discussion or feedback period. The first five weeks focused on exercising each limb consistently, while the last three weeks were devoted to practising the complete eight-limbed meditation. Participants were supplied with a meditation manual and an audio recording of guided commentary for self-practice. The intervention commenced for the first and second batches on 12 September 2022, and concluded on 10 November 2022. The third batch started its session on 3 October 2022, and wrapped up on 27 November 2022.

Intervention Technique

The investigators designed this intervention module to incorporate the eight limbs of the Yoga Sutra into a meditative form. They believed that incorporating the Yoga Sutra's guidelines into a meditative form would help individuals internalise the teachings of the Yoga Sutra into their daily lives. Therefore, they developed the activities to ensure the intervention was tailored to their needs.

Initiation: Initiation is not one of the eight limbs of the Yoga Sutra. It is merely intended to initiate the meditation session. Aum is mentioned in Indian philosophy and serves as the initiation of meditation. Aum Meditation is an excellent technique that concurrently revitalises the mind and body (Harne et al., 2019). It also possesses many therapeutic benefits, as Pothugunta and Babu (2020) indicated. Furthermore, this meditation technique relieves stress and anxiety and improves memory (Wani et al., 2020; Alpert, 2015).

Technique: Take a deep breath and, while you exhale entirely, say "AUM" as you finish. Divide the AUM syllable into the sounds A-A-U-U-M-M, pause, and visualise the white light inside the body. Then, repeat five times. Take a deep breath and relax completely.

The next step in the module is to practice the first two Limbs of Yoga, i.e., Yamas and Niyamas, where Yamas are the avoidance of immoral acts, and Niyamas are the performance of moral disciplines (Jain, 2022; Ram, 2010). The investigators used the tailored form of Rajyoga, and the meditative activities are described below.

Yamas

Ahimsa: Ahimsa is the act of non-violence, and to infuse the value of kindness, one must practise non-violence (Hughes, 2017). The more it is practised, the more peace, love, and compassion radiate from every action. To cultivate ahimsa, the exercise suggested by investigators is *Stop Check and Change:* Contemplate any event that disturbed you today or in the past week, any scene where you want to change your response. Visualise that scene again and see the flow of negative thoughts coming to the mind. Label the feelings, colour those feelings, and see that sensation in your body. Now Stop the flow of those thoughts and change, replace the colour of that emotion with a happy colour, and mentally transform negative responses into constructive ones. Visualise yourself crossing that same scene with a different response and colour. Take a deep breath and relax.

Satya: Satya means being honest and truthful. It is essential to uplift our consciousness and maintain an awareness of Purusha, which embodies the ultimate reality (Jain, 2022; Ram, 2010). The exercise suggested is *to reflect upon*: Direct your entire attention inward and disconnect from your physical surroundings and body. Reflect upon and speak in your mind … I am a spiritual energy … the embodiment of truth … I am the eternal soul … pure and potent … the master of this body … Focus on the center of the forehead and visualise the bright star there … visualise the layers of ignorance, untruth, and vices gently peeled off by waves of peace.

Asteya: Asteya means obtaining things through fair means and infusing the value of not stealing (Ram, 2010; Saraswati, 2009). The process of stealing is much more deceptive; it begins with cognition and ends with action. The exercise suggested is to *Practice Detachment* and rid yourself of all unnecessary desires. Reflect upon the possessions you have that are not yours and release the thoughts of holding or owning other's property.

Brahmacharya: Brahmacharya means leading a disciplined lifestyle and achieving the desired goals by cultivating self-control (Jain, 2022). The exercise suggested is to move beyond the Consciousness of the Body and practice redirecting attention. *Exercise-Inside Out:* Bring your entire focus inward, visualise a point of light inside your brain, experience the disconnection from the outside world, and feel your existence inside. After a short while, try to defocus by focusing solely outside your body and visualise the tip of your nose while also seeing the body from the outside. Feel the sensation of the outside environment and repeat.

Aparigraha: Aparigraha means not to possess. Possession of anything, including material goods, people, and status, eventually gives rise to feelings of attachment and pain (Jain, 2022; Ram, 2010). Suggested *Exercise: Bird Personification*: Choose a bird as your personification object. Imagine a bird (yourself) in the garden resting on a branch, and tag all the pointless thoughts on the branch, fear of losing something, attachment, dissatisfaction, anxiety; after a few seconds, flap your wings and fly away, high above the tree and letting go of every unnecessary desire. Feel as if you are a liberated bird, detached and free.

Niyamas

Saucha: The word Saucha means to keep your body and mind pure and clean (Jain, 2022). *The exercise* suggested for purifying one's mind is to visualise a lovely scene with a sky and clouds, where the clouds represent thoughts, and the sky represents a clear mind. Try to keep the sky as clear as you can; as the thoughts pass by, keep pushing them aside or letting them pass through the mind without judgement. Feel grateful when you get your mind clear.

Santosha: Santosha refers to satisfaction and contentment (Saraswati, 2009). Suggested *Exercise*: Inculcate contentment – Take a long, deep breath, breathe in peace and acceptance, and exhale out all the complaints and dissatisfaction that you have been holding in until now. Monitor your thoughts and imagine a red light of unconditional love and acceptance; continue passing this ball of red light to the people and things on your gratitude list. Breathe in acceptance and breathe out gratitude and love.

Tapas: Tapas means applying one's heart to a particular task to overcome all physical and mental obstacles (Ram, 2010). *Exercise*: Visualise a flame on your hand and feel its warmth and the tingling sensation it causes. Commit to yourself that you will tolerate any situation or any kind of difficulty and that you will keep going inside until you reach your goal.

Svadhyaya: Svadhyaya is a path to self-awareness or personal development; it is a study of oneself. The path determining your strengths and weaknesses, list them out and reflect and introspect upon them (Jain, 2022). *Exercise:* Take a deep breath and relax. It is time to introspect and know yourself more, scan your whole day, and introspect on what went wrong. Prepare for the next day, introspect on your strength, and embrace it more. Inhale peace and exhale out all negative emotions and feelings that do not serve you anymore.

Ishvara Pranidhana means supreme cosmic energy or supreme being, and pranidhana means to surrender (Jain, 2022). *Exercise*: Visualise a divine star before you brimming with divinity and bright light. Give all your worries, tensions, and fears to that divine star (Supreme power/God) that appears as light, and express gratitude for this beautiful life. Feel the lightness and charge as you are in the canopy of God.

Asana

The term 'asana' refers to a sitting position. There are two categories of asanas: corrective asanas and another is meditative asanas; in this intervention plan, the investigator has blended them. The Sage Patanjali did not specify any particular asana (Jain, 2022). Suggested Exercise: *Loosening Up Drill:* is the combination of self-made exercises listed below that are combined with physical exercises, some visualisation techniques, and affirmations. These are as follows:

Vision 360

Eyes Movements based on Nethra Sanchalana. Sit comfortably and rapidly blink your eyes a few times and move your eyes clockwise and anticlockwise, while doing the exercise practice affirmation (I am Happy Being). Repeat ten times with both eyes while visualising white light in the eyes. Rub your hands and put on your eyes.

Head-2-Shoulder

Neck Exercise based on Greeva Sanchalana. Sit comfortably and move your head clockwise and anticlockwise. Practice affirmation: "I am wonderful." Repeat ten times on both sides while visualising white light over the neck and feeling charged up.

Warmup Arms

Shoulder Rotation based on Skandha Chakra. Sit comfortably, put your hands on your shoulder, and practice the affirmation - I Am Powerful. While moving the arms Up and Down, practice affirmation - I Am Beautiful, and while rotating the arms, practice the affirmation - I Am Proud of Myself. Repeat 10 times with both arms while visualising white light in arms, feeling charged.

Elbow Bending is based on Kehuni Naman. Sit comfortably, stretch out your hands away from the body, and practice the affirmation "I am Strong or I am Loving." Repeat 10 times with both arms while visualising white light in your arms, feeling charged.

Hand Clenching based on Mushtika Bandhana. Sit comfortably, lift your hand to the shoulder level, open your fist completely, and tightly close the fist while closing the fingers with your thumb. Furthermore, visualise as if you are finishing all feelings of anger/hate by closing them tightly, and only peace remains in the palm. Repeat 10 times with both arms while visualising white light in the palm; feel charged.

Wrist Rotation based on Manibandha Chakra. Hold the fist and rotate without moving the elbow by making a circle clockwise and anticlockwise in each direction. Hold happiness and peace in the fist and rotate 10–15 times.

Wrist Bending based on Manibandha Naman. Open your palm, stretch your arms at shoulder level, and visualise light from the hand up and down, spreading peace and happiness to everyone around you. Do it 10–15 times and visualise the red light of blessings flowing through your palm.

Power Walk

Toe Bending based on Padanguli Naman. Sit comfortably and outstretch your legs with feet apart. Move the toes of both feet up and down. Hold for a few seconds and visualise the light all over your feet. Practice this 10–15 times, hold for a few seconds and visualise the light all over your feet.

Ankle Rotation based on Goolf Chakra. Sit comfortably with outstretched legs with both feet together and slowly rotate the ankle clockwise and anticlockwise. Practice detachment with the affirmation - I am a Guest on Earth. Practice this 10–15 times, hold for a few seconds, and visualise the light all over your feet.

Ankle Bending based on Goolf Naman. Sit comfortably by keeping your feet apart and moving your feet forward and backwards while you bend your feet forward; visualise all the negative feelings going out through the toes, and when you stretch inside, visualise the light of positivity going towards the body. Repeat 10 times while visualising white light all over and feel charged.

Outstretch: The Complete Stretch

While sitting in the base position, stretch your hands upward and inhale deeply. Visualise the universal power entering inside the body, bend forward, and hold for a few seconds. Once you are done, inhale back and sit straight. Repeat ten times while visualising white light all over your body, and feel charged.

You are now moving further, remaining still and silent. Place your legs crossed or folded in a comfortable position called a Meditative Pose. While doing further exercises, your other muscles/ asanas are Vajrasana, Padmasana, or Sukhasana.

Pranayama

Pranayama is the technique that allows one to control and energise the breath to reach a higher energy state. The exercise Suggested by the investigator here is *Rhythmic Breathing 1:1:1* based on Nadi Sodhana/Anuloma-Viloma Pranayama-Breathe in and out while seated in Padmasana or Sukhasana. Inhale deeply to fill your lungs with air from your left nostril while blocking your right nostril. Block your left nostril while holding your breath and exhale through the right nostril (Arya, 2017). Slow down the breath and the rhythm of 1:1:1 to be followed. Inhale all the positive energy (visualising white light), hold it in your body for a few seconds and feel it spreading all over the body. Then, exhale out completely, visualising detoxification of mind and body.

Pratyahara

Pratyahara is the practice of withdrawing one's attention from the senses, redirecting inward, and internalising it (Satchidananda, 2012). The mind has a significant impact on our entire life. Exercise Suggested is *Step In-Step Out*: Close your eyes and visualise the room/space holistically where you are currently sitting, for a few seconds and then step by step, keep moving inward and shift your attention to closer things; now step in more and focus on your body, and then after a few seconds move in further and focus inside the head on point of light, stay there for few seconds and gradually keep stepping out, from one point of the body to big picture of the room.

Dharana, Dhyana, and Samadhi

Dharana, Dhyana, and Samadhi are the three inner limbs, and they are known as Sanyam (control), or the path to the absolute light of knowledge, the journey of self-awareness (Jain, 2022). One can practice them all together as there is no dividing line between them. The exercise suggested by the investigator is *Centration-Point Concentration*: Dharna is the process of fixing the mind on a particular object or concept (soul or energy). By the repeated practice of focusing the mind on a particular object, it gradually develops into Dhyana, and the long stability of the mind develops in samadhi. *Exercise- Infinite Bliss*: Sit comfortably and relax … Breathe in and breathe out completely … visualise yourself as being of light (soul) and stabilise your attention on it … and visualise another point of light, i.e., supreme light … merge your consciousness with the supreme light/power … Feel the oneness and ultimate bliss … Om Shanti.

Silence: Silence after meditation is a way to bring awareness within and internalise the new experience. Maintain silence for one minute, and the inner journey ends.

Results

Data was analysed using descriptive statistics. A paired measure t-test was used to compare significant mean differences between the pre–post-assessment and the calculation of Cohen's.

Table 9.1 illustrates notable changes in the pre- and post-test scores of the intervention group. The anxiety subscale revealed a significant decrease in the post-assessment mean score (M=12.63) compared to the pre-assessment mean score (M=14.84). Similarly, the stress, depression, regression, fatigue, and guilt subscales showed a significant reduction in post-assessment scores compared to their respective pre-assessment scores. On the other hand, the extraversion and arousal subscales showed a significant increase in post-assessment scores compared to their pre-assessment scores. Significant t-ratios were found for anxiety (t=3.80; p<.01), stress (t=1.96; p<.05), depression (t=2.57; p<.05), regression (t=2.71; p<.01), fatigue (t=3.59; p<.01), guilt (t=3.39; p<.01), extraversion (t=–2.61; p<.05) and arousal (t=–3.58; p<.01), indicating that Rajyoga meditation has a significant effect on overall negative affect. The effect size for all subscales of negative affect, as determined by Cohen's d, showed a small effect. It includes a small effect size for the anxiety state (Cohen's d=.442), the stress state (Cohen's d=2.28), the depression state (Cohen's d=.299), the regression state (Cohen's d=.316), and the Fatigue state (Cohen's d=.417). The Guilt state also demonstrated a small effect size (Cohen's d=.394). The extraversion and arousal states also showed a small effect size (Cohen's d=–.304 and d=–.416, respectively; Figure 9.1).

Table 9.1 Results of Paired Samples *t*-test Analysis Examining the Role of the Intervention Technique on Negative Affect

Variables	Pre-assessment		Post-assessment		t (74)	p	Cohen's d
	M	SD	M	SD			
Anxiety	14.84	5.00	12.63	5.67	3.80	.000	.442
Stress	14.50	3.53	13.69	3.82	1.96	.050	.228
Depression	13.38	4.92	11.89	4.98	2.57	.012	.299
Regression	14.50	4.28	12.93	4.94	2.71	.008	.316
Fatigue	15.05	5.03	13.16	5.48	3.59	.001	.417
Guilt	13.48	4.72	11.78	5.14	3.39	.001	.394
Extraversion	21.40	4.04	22.66	4.10	2.61	.011	−.304
Arousal	19.78	4.52	21.45	4.75	3.58	.001	−.416

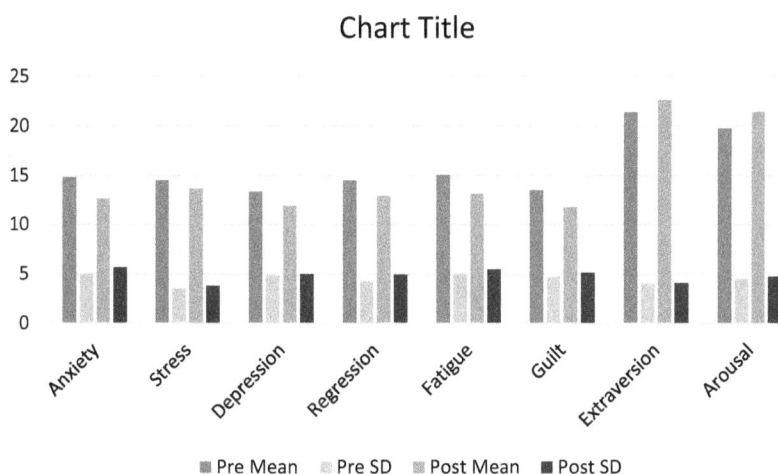

Figure 9.1 Mean and SD of Pre- and Post-Assessment.

Discussion

The intervention program of eight weeks led to a notable decrease in negative emotional states, such as anxiety, depression, regression, fatigue, and guilt. Further, there was a substantial change in the depression of the participants, indicating that rajyoga meditation reduces disappointment, pessimism, and dissatisfaction. Nonetheless, other indicators of negative affect, such as regression, fatigue, and guilt, showed a significant decrease in the post-assessment; participants were less confused, more organised, and had better concentration. They also reported feeling less tired throughout the day, less regretful about the past, and less dissatisfied with themselves. On the other hand, there was a notable increase in the participants' extraversion and arousal, suggesting that Raj Yoga meditation enhances alertness, sharpens senses, boosts enthusiasm, and improves social comfort. Current

results were consistent with previous research where it was found that yoga practice, including asana, pranayama, and meditation, alleviates negative affect like
stress, anxiety, depression, and fear (Madhu et al., 2022; Lemay et al., 2019; Saeed
et al., 2010), fatigue (Boehm et al., 2012), and guilt (Singh & Pandey, 2013) and
improves the overall health by strengthening the immunity of mind and body (Jain,
2020; Bushell et al., 2020; Boaventura et al., 2022). Findings from the study confirm the usefulness of various techniques that can be implemented in daily life.

Rajyoga meditation practised rigorously for at least 30 days enhanced psychological well-being and relieved the psychological crisis, stress, and anxiety that
occurred due to the COVID-19 pandemic (Madhu et al., 2022; Jain, 2020). Even
short-term Rajyoga meditation can positively impact psychological well-being
(Rasania, 2021) because the meditation's proficiency matters more than the duration of the session (Nair et al., 2018). It fosters connection and strengthens physical, mental, emotional, and spiritual wellness (Santos et al., 2023; Nagendra et al.,
2015) and is a way of living life to its fullest.

Meditation, yoga asanas (physical postures), and pranayama have all been suggested to deal with the pandemic's psychological distress (Sharp, 2020). Yoga,
now in the 20th century, is perceived as a therapeutic intervention (Khalsa et al.,
2016; Santos et al., 2023). It is a wholesome package for mental and physical wellness, regardless of gender, age, profession, or level of physical and mental health;
Rajyoga should be practised worldwide (Singh et al., 2021) as a means of leading a
healthy and prosperous life (Singh et al., 2011; Shaha & Gupta, 2018).

Conclusion

The results of this study suggested that Rajyoga meditation may be a helpful tool
for reducing negative affect if practised regularly. Numerous studies have suggested developing a therapy based on Sage Patanjali's Yoga Sutras (Chowdhary &
Gopinath, 2013; Balodhi & Chowdhary, 1986) for managing psychological issues.
Therefore, the researcher paved the way to introduce the intervention technique
incorporating all eight limbs of yoga in meditative form. The present study opens up
an avenue to utilise the potential of yogic philosophy as a complementary therapy.
It provides future directions to explore the effects of Rajyoga meditation on other
aspects of mental health. However, there are still very few general and adequate
strategies based on Patanjali Yoga Sutras specifically for COVID-19 crisis management. Rajyoga meditation has the potential to enhance mental wellness. Practising
the eight limbs together is recommended for a more holistic and comprehensive
approach. One limitation of the present study is the need for a control group and
lack of control over extraneous variables like family and financial circumstances.
Future research could validate the intervention using different methodologies and
apply it to diverse demographic and cultural contexts.

Acknowledgements

We sincerely thank all the participants who remained dedicated and consistent
throughout the intervention. Their cooperation and commitment were essential

to the study's data collection. Moreover, it was a delightful experience to interact with individuals from diverse backgrounds and understand their life experiences.

References

Alpert, Y. M. (2015). Mastering the Om: A guide for beginners. *Yoga Journal.* https://www.yogajournal.com/yoga-101/sanskrit/mastering om/

Araujo, R. V., Fernandes, A. F. C., Campelo, R. C. V., Silva, R. A., & Nery, I. S. (2021). Effect of raja yoga meditation on the distress and anxiety levels of women with breast cancer. *Religions, 12*(8), 590.

Arora, A. K., & Girgila, K. K. (2014). Effect of short-term Rajyoga meditation on anxiety and depression. *Pakistan Journal of Physiology, 10*(1–2), 18–20.

Arya, K. (2017). *Yoga education.* Daryaganj: Friends Publication.

Balodhi, J. P., & Chowdhary, J. R. (1986). Psychiatric concepts in Atharva Veda: A review. *Indian Journal of Psychiatry, 28*(1), 63–68.

Bhide, S. R., Bhargav, H., Varambally, S., & Desai, G. (2022). Coping with COVID-19: What can we learn from Patanjali Yoga Sutras. *Journal of Psychiatry Spectrum, 1*(2), 125–128.

Boaventura, P., Jaconiano, S., & Ribeiro, F. (2022). Yoga and Qigong for health: Two sides of the same coin? *Behavioral Sciences, 12*(7), 222.

Boehm, K., Ostermann, T., Milazzo, S., & Büssing, A. (2012). Effects of yoga interventions on fatigue: A meta-analysis. *Evidence-Based Complementary and Alternative Medicine, 2012*, 124703.

Braboszcz, C., Hahusseau, S., & Delorme, A. (2010). Meditation and neuroscience: From basic research to clinical practice. In R. Carlstedt (Ed.), *Integrative clinical psychology, psychiatry and behavioural medicine: Perspectives, practices and research* (pp. 1910–1929). Springer Publishing.

Bushell, W., Castle, R., Williams, M. A., Brouwer, K. C., Tanzi, R. E., Chopra, D., & Mills, P. J. (2020). Meditation and yoga practices as potential adjunctive treatment of SARS-CoV-2 infection and COVID-19: A brief overview of critical subjects. *The Journal of Alternative and Compleme* Table 9.1 Results of Paired Samples *t*-test Analysis Examining the Role of the Intervention Technique on Negative Affect *ntary Medicine, 26*(7), 547–556.

Chouhan, M., & Singh, V. (2021). A study of wellbeing among Rajyoga meditators and non-meditators. *Indian Journal of Positive Psychology, 12*(1), 14–15.

Chowdhary, S., & Gopinath, J. K. (2013). Clinical hypnosis and Patanjali yoga sutras. *Indian Journal of Psychiatry, 55*(Suppl. 2), S157.

Curran, J. P., & Cattell, R. B. (1976). *Eight state questionnaire (8SQ).* Champaign, IL: Institute for Personality and Ability Testing.

Harne, B. P., Tahseen, A. A., Hiwale, A. S., & Dhekekar, R. S. (2019). Survey on Om meditation: Its effects on the human body and Om meditation as a tool for stress management. *Psychological Thought, 12*(1).

Hughes, A. (2017). Ahimsa: The number one yama of the first limb of Yoga. *Yogapedia.*

Jain, D. (2020). A randomised trial to evaluate the effect of meditation on Stress and Anxiety due to COVID-19 in a healthy adult population. *Pesquisa.bvsalud.org.*

Jain, R. (2022). What is Raja Yoga? The Yoga of Physical and Mental Control. Arhantayoga. https://tinyurl.com/2s4hmyv4

Kiran, U., Ladha, S., Makhija, N., Kapoor, P. M., Choudhury, M., Das, S., ... & Airan, B. (2017). The role of Rajyoga meditation for modulation of anxiety and serum cortisol in patients undergoing coronary artery bypass surgery: A prospective randomized control study. *Annals of Cardiac Anaesthesia, 20*(2), 158.

Khalsa, S. B., Cohen, L., McCall, T., & Telles, S. (2016). *Principles and practice of Yoga in health care*. Jessica Kingsley Publishers, 11(1).

Latha, S. (2014). An approach to counselling based on the yoga sutra of Patanjali. *International Journal of Yoga and Applied Science, 3*(1), 5–11.

Lazar, S. W., Kerr, C. E., Wasserman, R. H., Gray, J. R., Greve, D. N., Treadway, M. T., & Benson, H. (2005). Meditation experience is associated with increased cortical thickness. *Neuroreport, 16*(17), 1893.

Lemay, V., Hoolahan, J., & Buchanan, A. (2019). Impact of a yoga and meditation intervention on students' stress and anxiety levels. *American Journal of Pharmaceutical Education, 83*(5), 7001.

Levine, G. N., Lange, R. A., Bairey-Merz, C. N., Davidson, R. J., Jamerson, K., Mehta, P. K., & American Heart Association Council; Council on Cardiovascular and Stroke Nursing; and Council on Hypertension. (2017). Meditation and cardiovascular risk reduction: A scientific statement from the American Heart Association. *Journal of the American Heart Association, 6*(10), e002218.

Madhu, S., Govindaraj, R., Kumar, P., & Chandra, S. (2022). Stress and the impact of stressful events are lesser among raja yoga meditators: A cross-sectional study during COVID-19 pandemic from India. *Clinical eHealth, 5*, 58–66.

Mayer, J. D. (2000). Spiritual intelligence or spiritual consciousness? *The International Journal for the Psychology of Religion, 10*(1), 47–56.

Nagendra, H., Kumar, V., & Mukherjee, S. (2015). Cognitive behaviour evaluation based on physiological parameters among young, healthy subjects with yoga as an intervention. *Computational and Mathematical Methods in Medicine, 2015*, 821061.

Nair, A. K., John, J. P., Mehrotra, S., & Kutty, B. M. (2018). What contributes to well-being gains–proficiency or duration of meditation-related practices? *International Journal of Wellbeing, 8*(2), 68–88.

Padhan, G. (2022). Spiritual psychotherapeutic healing post Covid-19: A novel approach in healthcare. *Computer Integrated Manufacturing Systems, 28*(10), 756–779.

Patel, N. (1996). Effect of Rajayoga Meditation in treating neurotic illnesses and changes in physiological parameters. *GHRC Bulletin*.

Pizer, A. (2023). Yoga sutras of Patanjali: The 8 limbs of Yoga explained. *Lifeform*.

Pothugunta, S., & Babu, K. R. (2020). Significance of Om meditation in classical Yoga texts and its therapeutic benefits. *Journal of Critical Reviews, 7*(1).

Prabhavananda, S., & Isherwood, C. (1948). *Patanjali yoga sutras: Translated with a new commentary* (pp. 17–19). Chennai: Sri Ramakrishna Math.

Pulla, P. (2020). COVID-19: India imposed lockdown for 21 days, and cases rose. *British Medical Journal, 368*, 1251.

Ram, B. (2010). *The eight limbs of Yoga – pathway to liberation*. New Delhi: Motilal Banarsidass Publishers Private Limited.

Rao, N. G. (2012). *Patanjali's Ashtanga Yoga & human life*.

Rasania, S. K. (2021). A cross-sectional study of mental wellbeing with practice of yoga and meditation during COVID-19 pandemic. *Journal of Family Medicine and Primary Care, 10*(4), 1576.

Satchidananda, S. (2012). *The yoga sutras of patanjali: Translation and commentary by Sri Swami Satchidananda*. Buckingham, VA: Integral Yoga Publications.

Saeed, S. A., Antonacci, D. J., & Bloch, R. M. (2010). Exercise, yoga, and meditation for depressive and anxiety disorders. *American Family Physician, 81*(8), 981–986.

Santos, D. C., Jaconiano, S., Macedo, S., Ribeiro, F., Ponte, S., Soares, P., & Boaventura, P. (2023). Yoga for COVID-19: An ancient practice for a new condition – a literature review. *Complementary Therapies in Clinical Practice, 50,* 101717.

Saraswati, S. S. (2009). *Asana pranayama mudra bandha.* Munger, Bihar, India: Yoga Publication Trust.

Satsangi, A. K., & Brugnoli, M. P. (2018). Anxiety and psychosomatic symptoms in palliative care: From neuro-psychobiological response to stress to symptoms' management with clinical hypnosis and meditative states. *Annals of Palliative Medicine, 7*(1), 75–111.

Sekhsaria, K. P. (2020). *How Hindu spiritual practices can help manage your COVID-19 anxiety.* Hinduamerican.org.

Shaha, R., & Gupta, S. (2018). Role of Rajyoga meditation as psychotherapy in various physical and mental illnesses and wellbeing. *Indian Journal of Positive Psychology, 9*(1), 114–116.

Shanker, S., Sadhana, S., Lal, B., Agarwal, G., & Bute, J. (2018). Study to evaluate the impact of Rajyoga meditation on psychosomatic aspects of hypertensive patients. *Journal of Medical Science and Clinical Research, 6*(11). https://doi.org/10.18535/jmscr/v6i11.81.

Sharp, J. (2020). *Coping with coronavirus anxiety.* Harvard Health Blog. Harvard Health Publishing.

Singh, A., Sharma, S. B., Rana, A., Amandeep, K., Kaur, A., & Rani, B. (2021). Effectiveness of Rajyoga Meditation: A quasi-experimental study for holistic healing in cancer patients. *Environment Conservation Journal, 22*(1&2), 35–40.

Singh, B., & Pandey, S. (2013). Spiritual healing and Rajyoga Meditation in schizo affective disorder, depressive type: A case report. *International Journal of Science and Research (IJSR), 14*(6), 2319–7064.

Singh, S., Mohan, M., & Kumar, R. (2011). Enhancing physical health, psychological health, and emotional intelligence through Sahaj Marg Raj yoga meditation practice. *Indian Journal of Psychological Science, 2,* 89–98.

Varambally, S., & Gangadhar, B. N. (2012). Yoga: A spiritual practice with therapeutic value in psychiatry. *Asian Journal of Psychiatry, 5*(2), 186–189.

Wani, L. K., Upasani, D. E., & Deshpande, A. (2020, November). Review of scientific analysis of sacred sound Om (Aum). *JETER, 7*(11).

WHO. (2022, March 2). *COVID-19 pandemic triggers a 25% increase in the prevalence of anxiety and depression worldwide.* WHO.

Yogeshwar, G. (1994). Swami Vivekananda's concept of jnana yoga, raja yoga, karma yoga and bhakti yoga. *Ancient Science of Life, 13*(3–4), 261.

10 A Critical Study

The Transactional Concept of Coping through Electronic Media during the COVID-19 Pandemic

Sruthi Suresh, Abhay Rabia, and A.V. Abirami

Introduction

Grief and Coping

Human life is filled with many ups and downs, and no one can expect to remain in a constant state of emotion. Grief is one such emotion which every human being tries to avoid, but eventually, each will have at least a few encounters with it. Grief as an emotion is a painful and almost universal human experience caused by a wide range of physiological and psychological factors (Averill, 1968). Grief comes in many types. Anticipatory grief happens when one anticipates an actual loss before it happens (Aldrich, 1974). Abbreviated grief occurs when one gets over the grief phase faster than usual. This kind of grief usually happens after anticipatory grief. Thus, all the cognitive heavy lifting regarding the loss is already done before the actual loss occurs, and once the loss occurs, the individual copes with the grief faster (Vasquez, 2021). Cumulative grief happens when an individual faces multiple miseries simultaneously (Team, 2021). Delayed grief happens when the loss that causes grief has passed, but the element of grief has not happened to the individual. The episode of suffering in this scenario occurs sometime after the loss (Rowe, 2022). Inhibited grief occurs at certain times when individuals repress their emotions of grief after the event of loss (Krull, 2022).

These are a few kinds of grief that individuals manifest when going through a phase of loss. People try to deal with these episodes of distress in unique ways. 'Coping' is how people deal with such stages of loss and ensuing grief. It is usually defined as the process of adjusting or tolerating adverse events. At the same time, one strives to keep a positive outlook regarding one's life and maintain one's emotional stability (Chowdhury, 2019). As the element of stress is unique for each individual, the methods they use to cope with these stressors are also unique. Some may adopt more constructive coping mechanisms, such as developing a new hobby or indulging themselves in their favourite work to overcome stress. On the other hand, some are inclined towards adopting harmful coping mechanisms, such as smoking and drinking, in order to mitigate the effect of the stress caused by grief.

DOI: 10.4324/9781003454984-11

Stages of Grief and Bereavement

There are multiple stages to grief, as per the Kubler-Ross model (2014) (DABDA). It is postulated that a person in grief goes through the five stages of denial, anger, bargaining, depression, and acceptance (Feldman, 2017). In the denial stage, the individual has not accepted the fact that he is faced with a situation in which he has to deal with grief. It could be anything ranging from the diagnosis of a terminal illness to the death of a near one. In the second stage of anger, the individual accepts that he or she cannot always stay in denial, which would frustrate them. This frustration leads to anger, where they try to find reasons why they were the ones to be in this situation or who was the reason for them to be in this situation. The third stage is the stage of bargaining, where the individual tries to find ways to avoid facing grief by trying to find ways around it. In the fourth stage, the stage of depression, the individuals, when they see that they cannot avoid grief in any manner, they usually go into a state of depression. Finally, at the fifth stage, they accept that the grief they are facing is unavoidable, and the only way out of this situation is to face it. Recently, 'meaning' or finding meaning is also seen as the sixth stage of grief (Kessler, 2019). In all these stages, individuals usually adopt different coping mechanisms.

Types of Coping

Individuals attempt to cope with grief through multiple methods. In the early stages of research into various coping strategies, Lazarus and Folkman (1987) developed four prominent strategies individuals use to cope. They were problem-focused coping, emotion-focused coping, support-focused coping, and meaning-making coping (Folkman & Moskowitz, 2004). In current times, types of coping strategies are broadly bundled under the following categories.

- **Appraisal-focused coping** in which individuals going through grief usually alter their perception regarding grief in order to mitigate the stress that they experience from that grief. Individuals deliberately change their views on grief to get a more positive outlook (Senanayake et al., 2018).
- **Emotion-focused coping,** in which the focus is on managing the emotions that arise due to the stress caused by grief (Brannon & Feist, 2009). Releasing one's pent-up emotions, distracting oneself, and mindfulness practices are all different strategies that come under this broad coping strategy.
- **Reactive and proactive coping**, whereas most coping strategies are usually reactive. One undertakes a coping strategy once he or she is faced with a stressor. When one anticipates the occurrence of a stressor and adopts a coping mechanism in advance, seeing the advent of a stressor in future is called proactive coping (Brannon & Feist, 2009).
- **Social coping** is when the individual takes help from societal elements, such as social support systems, to overcome their stressors.

Individual Experiences of Grief and Coping during the COVID-19 Pandemic

At the end of the months of 2019, the world did not know that the coming year would bring about one of the most devastating pandemics that humanity has faced in about a century. By the end of 2021, the pandemic had claimed the lives of around 5.4 million people worldwide (Rigby, 2022) and had caused an international lockdown on human movement and migration. In essence, the entire world came to a grinding standstill. All these factors made the past two years the most stressful years that humankind had to persevere.

Grief came in various ways in these trying times, for example, the loss of a dear one, prolonged alienation from each other, and lack of social interaction. All could be seen as a stressor that causes grief. Since grief manifested in different ways during COVID-19, people also adopted unique coping mechanisms during these times. Losses in COVID-19 could be categorised into two types. The primary losses involved the death of someone near or any other loss that left a substantial impact on someone's mental health. The secondary losses stemmed from the impact left by the primary losses, such as a sense of loneliness due to the death of a near one (Zhai & Du, 2020).

One study found that increasing the sense of connectedness with nature (even virtually) decreased stress levels in young adults (Yeung & Yu, 2022). Community-specific coping style, where an individual finds relief from their stress by interacting with community factors, such as friends and relatives, was found to have influenced the coping strategies of individuals during the pandemic times (Duan & Zhu, 2020). Since person-to-person physical interactions were severely restricted during these times, social media platforms, such as WhatsApp and Facebook, were extensively used. The chapter attempts to review how individuals used media as a coping mechanism during COVID-19 to ease the grief they felt as they went through different stages of grief.

Conceptual Framework

The transactional model of coping proposed by Lazarus and Folkman (1987) outlines a four-stage development of stress, acknowledging the role of behavioural and cognitive responses to the situation (Goldstein et al., 2019). In the first stage of primary appraisal, an individual assesses the situation to know if it is relevant or irrelevant and a challenge or a threat. If the situation is considered a threat, the secondary appraisal occurs when the individual's coping ability is evaluated based on the situational demands and perceived resources. If the situational demands outweigh the perceived resources, then the individual experiences stress and begin engaging in coping strategies. In problem-focused coping, people take it upon themselves to see the situation as a problem and find ways to overcome it; however, in emotion-focused coping, people strive to manage the emotions that are felt in response to the stressor (Lazarus & Folkman, 1987). Some parts of this model have been tested and supported by empirical evidence, as reported by previous research studies (Obbarius et al., 2021). According to Pestonjee (1992, as cited in Romas &

Sharma, 2022), the model aligns with Eastern ideas of *Samkhya-yoga*. It states that stress is caused by *avidya* or faulty reality testing of self-appraisal (*asmita*), object appraisal (*raga*), threat appraisal (*dvesha*), or coping (*abhinivesha*).

Applying this theory to the present examination, when a person finds themselves in a situation that instils stress in them, for instance, grief due to the loss of a dear one, they at first do a cognitive appraisal of the situation. They try to give meaning to the situation and seek ways to cope.

Individuals who choose problem-focused coping strategies may use online resources and keep track of news reports and statistics or read blogs and websites to prepare for the situation (Chung & Kim, 2008). In emotion-focused coping, an individual finds a method to tackle the stressor emotionally. Mainly in this coping style, individuals either resort to avoiding or running away from emotionally tackling the stressor or trying to find emotional support from internal or external sources to cope with the stressor. Social media apps and other online entertainment media could provide an escape window out of stress-inducing situations by exposing them to content that lifts their mood by making them momentarily forget about the stressor (Nabi et al., 2022). The same media or content can sometimes aid in problem-focused and emotion-focused coping (Prestin & Nabi, 2020; Wolfers & Schneider, 2021). During COVID, prominent conventional media sources, such as television and radio started broadcasting self-help content in expert interviews to guide individuals in managing grief and stress and morale-boosting programs, such as spiritual talks and discussions.

Review of Literature

Role of Electronic Media as a Coping Mechanism

The Lazarus and Folkman concept reflects stress, the bond between a person and the environment regarded as highly meaningful and as straining or surpassing coping resources. This lens focuses on the importance of two ways: one is appraisal, and another is to cope as mediators (Folkman, 2013). This chapter exemplifies the coping idea used by Folkman and explains how, during COVID-19, humans used social media applications to reduce stress and overcome it. Isolation, lockdown, stress, low-key state, quarantine, and restricted social gatherings have pushed humans to use social media. Since social gatherings were shut down during the quarantine period, this phase saw the emergence of virtual gatherings. This phase also witnessed the highest amount of stress and depression. To avoid this, instead of meeting people in larger social gatherings, it was shifted to expanding the followers list and increasing screen time. People's networking skills have shifted to online networking skills, which had an impact on mental health to a greater extent (Orsolini et al., 2022).

From passing on oral narration and stories to All India Radio and Doordarshan, from trusted sources people rely on, the media industry has undergone tremendous change. The relationship between media and its demographic audiences is described as authentic and promising. It articulates truth, declares fragile information, and is meant for entertainment.

On the other hand, television has a larger audience despite the age group one belongs to. Television media provides unlimited content for its audience, from which one can choose which channel and content to view. For instance, the channels meant only for comedy, music, movies, and kids' cartoons have tremendously increased as everyone faces lockdowns (Arend et al., 2021).

In contrast to the above example, news channel rates and TRP have increased as the pandemic was considered a national emergence and viewers kept track of death rates and rise. Like cause and effect, people were pushed to stress, anxiety, and mental health, and a low-key state media industry served as an easily accessible escape. The primary reasons one tends to use media are to overcome emotional fear and family member loss, get rid of stress, equip oneself, get rid of boredom, overcome layoffs, and do courses. People were eager to search on the internet for expanding cases of COVID-19 and to fetch updates on death rate cases through the news media during the early stages of COVID-19. Similarly, misinformation and misleading news guidance were being passed on the internet, which had a negative impact on the human self (Ferreria Caceres et al., 2022). For example, the usage of dating apps avoided suicidal thoughts for youngsters who were facing the breakup stage; this bridged the gap between traditional dating. Online dating eradicates perceived loneliness and decreases the stress of safety in communicating with strangers through the application; these apps provide a text-friendly platform and help to cope with rejection since it is online (Ann et al., 2020).

Additionally, broadcasts and podcasts are audio versions without videos; this incorporates television, digital radio, and experts of particular fields discussing sensitive issues and recording audio about unique topics that assist visually impaired listeners and clarify the obscure. Electronic media consists of sources and information that can be accessed online; it also includes study materials, journal articles, and even e-newspapers; e-books are available. Internet media is slightly different from electronic media; it incorporates social media applications, such as YouTube and OTT platforms that have seen the utmost growth in the media world. Watching, reading, maintaining sleep, and health tracking apps were seen as an escape from the chaos. Human beings realised the importance of health and life during the pandemic, for which the media mentioned above served as a relaxing tool. It was cost-efficient for people to access media; some people used social media platforms to escape from reality.

Electronic Media Usage during COVID-19 Pandemic

Media usage builds a stronger foundation for demographic audiences in the era of artificial intelligence and satellites. The internet holds more credit for the rise of media with the advancement of technology. The media world presents more than precise information; however, it can assist people all over the globe in coping with adverse situations. The pandemic has made everyone strong and independent in their own ways through media. During the COVID-19 Pandemic, people faced lots of stress; they were put under a lot of emotional and mental trauma. Many families had lost their close ones during the pandemic, which significantly impacted them to continue their lives. The media played a vital role in coping despite age groups for one to cope with their schedule. Social media and screen time have become a comfortable space during uncertain situations. A study conducted on the role of media and its impact on the public stated that as a result, it was found that usage of television and the internet was at its peak during the pandemic. Few social media applications, such as YouTube, Instagram, OTT, and music applications gave hope and helped one move on with life.

Social media use made a home more comfortable for people who felt isolated; similarly, working from home online has drawn attention. Online yoga classes, High-intensity interval training sessions, and Zumba dance were major media for connecting with people. Switching from WhatsApp calling for office purposes has traditionally shifted to Microsoft, Google Meet, WebEX, Zoom and Twitter, which were seen as official means of communication. As publication houses were down, authors conducted online conferences. They invited participants from around the globe to be part of them, and teachers and friends conducted reading rooms in Zoom to mend the gap. The traditional classes were replaced with online space rooms via Google Classroom. Through this, the family did not just cope with the situation but simultaneously learned and started engaging with the applicants to connect with family members across the globe to bridge the gap. The audience felt it was beneficial to use the YouTube application as it assists one with revenge based on watching time and view, considering using time productively, exploring new talent, and serving good content for their consumers. Thus, several media types help one cope with mental health and well-being.

Electronic Media as Problem-Focused and Emotion-Focused Coping Mechanism

The media industry has a strong influence when it comes to coping as it offers a multi-dimensional shift for its audience. As several deaths had been encountered and witnessed by family members and close ones, the loss had a significant impact on people; thus, all types of media performed their best to help each other gear up as people faced. When social distancing was implemented, the level of anxiety in humans increased to subside this for kids and college students; schools and teachers learned the importance of mental health and conducted online and live classes for students. Heading towards the next level, universities organised live art and cultural competitions to improve students' health. Similarly, to support co-workers' and employees' state of mind, the office and management organised open cultural activities to reduce stress for their employees, which involved the participation of family members. Perhaps this duration was considered the hobby cheering phase, a bittersweet stage; for instance, parents had more opportunities to spend time with their kids and help them improve their studies.

Moreover, many were encouraged to articulate their experience of the vaccine's feelings and the after-effects, all explored on social media platforms. Due to the implementation of lockdowns worldwide with restrictions to be followed, OTT performed massive support as movies/ web series brought a shift from the current fear on Instagram, where influencers motivated people to normalise the situation and suggested precautionary measures with home remedies.

The pandemic was where every human being chose to create their style of innovation with the assistance of the media. Especially during this period when hashtags, such as celebrate the imperfection, perfectly perfect, get well soon, and recover were on trend (Landsberg, 2021). The music gradually helped people to cope with emotional stress, even for budding artists. For a person who prefers music to books, music applications, such as Spotify, iMusic, JioSaavan, Amazon Music, and Wynk Music have millions of users and listeners.

Discussion

A study done on 254 Canadian families on the digital screen time trends during COVID-19 found that there was a 74%, 61%, and 87% increase in screen time spent by mothers, fathers, and children, respectively, in comparison to pre-COVID trends (Carroll et al., 2020). Similar studies in Poland and China have also reported increased screen time among the studied individuals during COVID-19 (Hu et al., 2020; Górnicka et al., 2020). These trends point fingers towards the fact that digital media was seen to drastically increase in its usage among individuals during the pandemic. The increased use was to help individuals cope with stressors, such as isolation, misinformation and time wastage, work-life disruption, and personal loss (Figure 10.1).

Different aspects of the media, such as apps and online platforms, enabled media-based coping. The following paragraphs discuss each of the stressors and the respective media used to cope.

Interpersonal interaction, such as dating, was an essential social element hindered during the pandemic. Digital media was one gateway that allowed individuals to reduce the ensuing stress. Dating apps were extensively used during the COVID-19 period for finding romantic companionship. On 2 March 2020, when most of the world was initiating lockdowns, Tinder, a dating app, broke its record for the largest single-day activity with around 3 billion swipes. Even the conversation lengths on Tinder showed a 32% increase during this period, indicating that individuals used such dating apps to initiate meaningful conversations with others (Tinder, 2021).

Worldwide lockdown and almost complete standstill of day-to-day activities for an individual resulted in an increased amount of time at the hands of people. The increased availability of time also increased the stress of using it judiciously and not wasting the same. Digital media, such as online learning platforms, provided a convenience for this predicament. Individuals could use the excess time that they have with them to learn new skills and talents, as is corroborated by statistics. Coursera, an online learning platform, had 35 million registered users in 2018, which increased to 44 million by 2019 (9 million increase). In 2020, at the advent of COVID-19, it registered around 27 million new users, totalling 71 million (Wood, 2022). The increase in registered users for the e-learning platform has recently been unprecedented. Similar trends were seen in course enrollments, too.

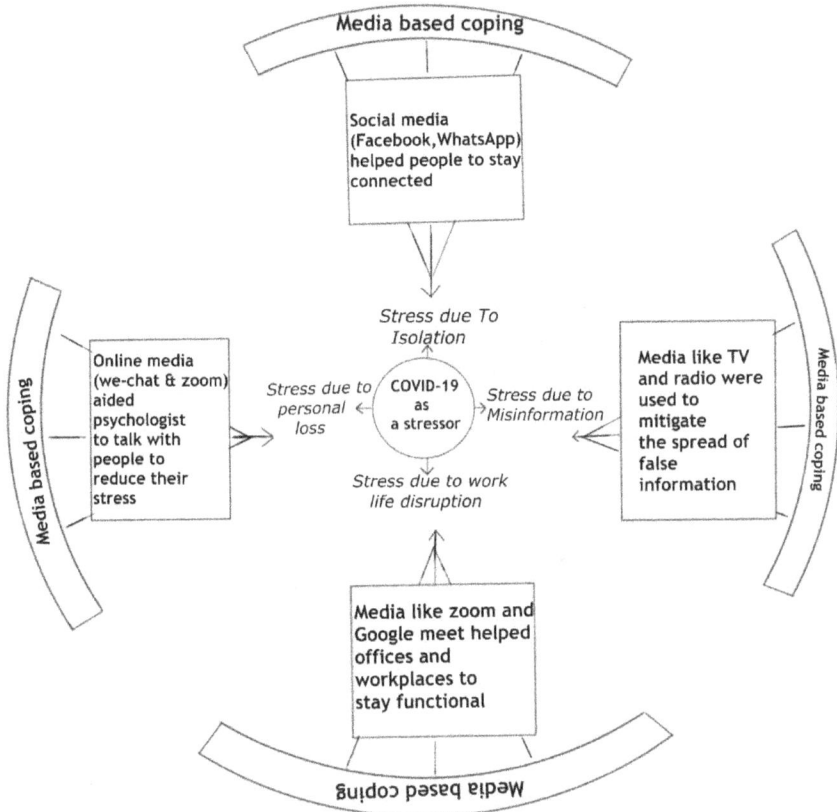

Figure 10.1 Different Forms of Stress during COVID-19 and How Media-based Coping Helped in Mitigating Them.

In 2019, Coursera had around 76 million course enrollments, skyrocketing to 143 million in 2020 (Wood, 2022).

The rampant spread of misinformation was also a cause of increasing stress among individuals. It is also important to note that constant media viewing related to disasters also affects individuals (Plude, 1992). Media helped mitigate the stress arising from the misinformation, too. Programs, such as 'Stop the Spread' were telecasted on popular media platforms, such as BBC World Television, website, and Apps in May and June 2020 to curb the spread of misinformation (WHO, 2021). Thus, in this manner, media became an effective coping mechanism that individuals worldwide adopted during the pandemic.

The work-life of individuals was also drastically affected during this period. The usual working style of being physically present at the workplace from morning till evening, was now suddenly impossible. Work is a significant part of an adult's life, and its sudden discontinuation is bound to act as a stressor in their life. Online media, such as Zoom and Google Meet have also become essential tools in mitigating stress levels. With the advent of new working styles, such as 'work-from-home', online platforms, such as Zoom became the need of the hour. These online media became an alternative bridge that connected individuals with their work lives. A study even said a 360% increase had been seen in using the Zoom platform during COVID-19 compared to pre-pandemic levels (Williams, 2021).

Similarly, the complete global lockdown during the pandemic negatively affected the education system worldwide. The risk of losing an academic year to the pandemic and its repercussions on their children's lives worried parents and primary guardians worldwide. Online media, such as Google Meet and Zoom lent a helping hand in reducing the stress caused by this fear. Teaching became online during the pandemic. An educational paradigm shift was seen during the pandemic when online modes of education replaced face-to-face classes through platforms, such as Zoom (Stefanile, 2020).

Finally, some individuals also experienced a personal loss of loved ones, which was one of the major stressors of the COVID times that created immense mental stress on individuals. Online mental help platforms came up to mitigate the increasing stress levels in society. A study conducted in China found that many mental health institutions had set up their online-based mental health services in digital media platforms, such as WeChat, to help people cope with stress (Liu et al., 2020). Psychology professionals use online media platforms, such as Zoom and WhatsApp to lend their expertise in mitigating the increasing stress levels in society. In contrast, Psychology professionals use online media platforms, such as Zoom and WhatsApp (Ifdil et al., 2020). According to Nabi et al. (2022), only TV/movie and music consumption emerged as a significant mediator between stress and coping efficacy.

Further research indicated that individuals also used social media to grieve by writing blogs and posting anecdotes about the deceased individual (Spiti et al., 2022). Individuals are also seen to create and maintain pages of the deceased persons as a space for collective grief and expression of continued care. However, the norms of virtual mourning and associated practices are still developing (Lingel, 2013).

Conclusion

There are several types of grief: anticipatory, abbreviated, cumulative, delayed, and inhibited grief. When crucial times like the pandemic arrived, almost everyone got lost, and it was solely the media industry that reconnected with each other. This research addresses restructured media usage and how people have adopted it as a coping mechanism. Transactional coping theory is utilised in the chapter with the application of Lazarus and Folkman (1987). The different stages of coping are appraisal-focused coping strategy, emotion-focused coping strategy, reactive and proactive coping strategy, and social coping.

During the COVID-19 pandemic, there was an increase in media usage among individuals. Based on a review of existing research, media-based coping was used for a range of stressors, including isolation, misinformation and time wastage, work-life disruption, and personal loss. It indicates a potential source of readily available, accessible, and effective coping which can be further explored. Such media-based coping strategies can be harnessed to support the rising number of individuals whose mental health needs cannot be catered to by the limited number of qualified mental health professionals. It can also be used to override the taboo that prevents individuals from seeking out support to cope with their stressors. Researchers and practising mental health professionals can explore the utility of media-based coping mechanisms and formulate plans to use them effectively.

Limitations

The present study reviews existing literature to contrast evidence and identify the research gaps but does not contribute empirical data or findings. The sources were selected according to the authors' discretion rather than based on any criteria or systematic process; hence, sources could have been missed or excluded. Media as a means of coping was the only concept explored; however, media could also negatively impact the individual or lead to problems, such as addiction, which were not explored in this study.

Acknowledgement

We are grateful to our families and friends for their support.

References

Aldrich, C. K. (1974). Some dynamics of anticipatory grief. In B. Schoenberg, A. C. Carr, D. Peretz, & A. H. Kutscher (Eds.), *Anticipatory grief* (pp. 1–4). New York: Columbia University Press.

Ann, M., Joshi, G., Rais, S., & Mishra, I. (2020, December 22). *Online dating: A motivated behaviour during pandemic*. Unknown. https://www.researchgate.net/publication/353378500_Online_dating_A_motivated_behavior_during_pandemic

Arend, A. K., Blechert, J., Pannicke, B., & Reichenberger, J. (2021). Increased screen use on days with increased perceived COVID-19 related confinements – A day level ecological momentary assessment study. *Frontiers in Public Health, 8*, 623205. https://doi.org/10.3389/fpubh.2020.623205

Averill, J. R. (1968). Grief: Its nature and significance. *Psychological Bulletin, 70*(6p1), 721.

Brannon, L., & Feist, J. (2009). Personal coping strategies. *Health psychology: An introduction to behaviour and health* (7th ed., pp. 121–123). Boston: Wadsworth Cengage Learning.

Carroll, N., Sadowski, A., Laila, A., Hruska, V., Nixon, M., Ma, D. W. L., Haines, J., & On Behalf of the Guelph Family Health Study. (2020). The impact of COVID-19 on health behaviour, stress, financial and food security among middle to high-income Canadian families with young children. *Nutrients, 12*(8), 2352. https://doi.org/10.3390/nu12082352

Chowdhury, M. R. (2019, September 3). *What is coping theory? Definition & worksheets*. Positive Psychology. Retrieved November 15, 2023, from https://positivepsychology.com/coping-theory/

Chung, D. S., & Kim, S. (2008). Blogging activity among cancer patients and their companions: Uses, gratifications, and predictors of outcomes. *Journal of the American Society for Information Science and Technology, 59*(2), 297–306. https://doi.org/10.1002/asi.20751

Duan, L., & Zhu, G. (2020). Psychological interventions for people affected by the COVID-19 epidemic. *The Lancet Psychiatry, 7*(4), 300–302. https://doi.org/10.1016/S2215-0366(20)30073-0

Ferreira Caceres, M. M., Sosa, J. P., Lawrence, J. A., Sestacovschi, C., Tidd-Johnson, A., Rasool, M. H. U., Gadamidi, V. K., Ozair, S., Pandav, K., Cuevas-Lou, C., Parrish, M., Rodriguez, I., & Fernandez, J. P. (2022). The impact of misinformation on the COVID-19 pandemic. *AIMS Public Health, 9*(2), 262–277. https://doi.org/10.3934/publichealth.2022018

Feldman, D. B. (2017). Why the five stages of grief are wrong. *Psychology Today*.

Folkman, S. (2013, January 1). *Stress: Appraisal and coping*. New York: Springer. https://link.springer.com/referenceworkentry/10.1007/978-1-4419-1005-9_215

Folkman, S., & Moskowitz, J. T. (2004). Coping: Pitfalls and promises. *Annual Review of Psychology, 55*(1), 745–774. https://doi.org/10.1146/annurev.psych.55.090902.141456

Goldstein, G., Allen, D. N., & deLuca, J. (2019). *Handbook of psychological assessment* (4th ed.). Cambridge: Academic Press. https://doi.org/10.1016/C2014-0-01970-3

Górnicka, M., Drywień, M. E., Zielinska, M. A., &Hamułk, J. (2020). Dietary and lifestyle changes during COVID-19 and the subsequent lockdowns among Polish adults: A cross-sectional online survey PLifeCOVID-19 study. *Nutrients, 12*(8). https://doi.org/10.3390/nu12082324

Hu, Z., Lin, X., Kaminga, A. C., & Xu, H. (2020). Impact of the COVID-19 epidemic on lifestyle behaviours and their association with subjective well-being among the general population in Mainland China: Cross-sectional study. *Journal of Medical Internet Research, 22*(8), e21176. https://doi/org/10.2196/21176

Ifdil, I., Fadli, R. P., Suranata, K., Zola, N., & Ardi, Z. (2020). Online mental health services in Indonesia during the COVID-19 outbreak. *Asian Journal of Psychiatry, 51*, 102153.

Kessler, D. (2019). *Finding meaning: The sixth stage of grief*. New York: Scribner.

Krull, E. (2022, May 31). *What's inhibited grief? And how does it work?* Joincake. Retrieved November 15, 2023, from https://www.joincake.com/blog/inhibited-grief/

Landsberg, T. (2021, July 28). How music helped during the pandemic? *Deutsche Welle*. https://www.dw.com/en/how-music-helped-during-the-pandemic/a-58668728

Lazarus, R. S., & Folkman. S. (1987). Transactional theory and research on emotions and coping. *European Journal of Personality, 1*(3), 141–169. https://doi.org/10.1002/per.2410010304

Lingel, J. (2013). The digital remains: Social media and practices of online grief. *The Information Society, 29*(3), 190–195. https://doi.org/10.1080/01972243.2013.777311

Liu, S., Yang, L., Zhang, C., Xiang, Y. T., Liu, Z., Hu, S., & Zhang, B. (2020). Online mental health services in China during the COVID-19 outbreak. *The Lancet Psychiatry, 7*(4), e17–e18.

Nabi, R. L., Wolfers, L. N., Walter, N., & Qi, L. (2022). Coping with COVID-19 stress: The role of media consumption in emotion- and problem-focused coping. *Psychology of Popular Media, 11*(3), 292–298. https://doi.org/10.1037/ppm0000374

Obbarius, N., Fischer, F., Liegl, G., Obbarius, A., & Rose, M. (2021). A modified version of the transactional stress concept according to Lazarus and Folkman, was confirmed in a psychosomatic inpatient sample. *Frontiers in Psychology, 12*. https://doi.org/10.3389/fpsyg.2021.584333

Orsolini, L., Volpe, U., Albert, U., Carmassi, C., Carrà, G., Cirulli, F., Dell'Osso, B., Del Vecchio, V., Di Nicola, M., Giallonardo, V., Luciano, M., Menculini, G., Nanni, M. G.,

Pompili, M., Sani, G., Sampogna, G., Tortorella, A., & Fiorillo, A. (2022). Use of social network as a coping strategy for depression among young people during the COVID-19 lockdown: Findings from the COMET collaborative study. *Annals of General Psychiatry, 21*(1), 44. https://doi.org/10.1186/s12991-022-00419-w

Plude, F. F. (1992). *Coping with disaster: How media audiences process grief.* Religion Online. https://www.religion-online.org/article/coping-with-disaster-how-media-audiences-process-grief/

Prestin, A., & Nabi, R. (2020). Media prescriptions: Exploring the therapeutic effects of entertainment media on stress relief, illness symptoms, and goal attainment. *Journal of Communication, 70*(2), 145–170. https://doi.org/10.1093/joc/jqaa001

Rigby, J. (2022). Almost three times as many died as a result of COVID than officially reported – WHO. *Reuters.*

Romas, J. A., & Sharma, M. (2022). *Practical stress management: A comprehensive workbook* (8th ed.). Academic Press. https://doi.org/10.1016/C2021-0-00818-X

Rowe, S. (2022, March 1). *Delayed grief: Causes, symptoms, and how to cope.* PsychCentral. Retrieved November 15, 2023, from https://psychcentral.com/health/delayed-grief

Senanayake, S., Harrison, K., Lewis, M., McNarry, M., & Hudson, J. (2018). Patients' experiences of coping with Idiopathic Pulmonary Fibrosis and their recommendations for its clinical management. *PLoS ONE, 13*(5), e0197660. https://doi.org/10.1371/journal.pone.0197660

Spiti, J. M., Davies, E., McLeish, P., & Kelly, J. (2022). How social media data are being used to research the experience of mourning: A scoping review. *PLoS ONE, 17*(7), e0271034. https://doi.org/10.1371/journal.pone.0271034

Stefanile, A. (2020). The transition from classroom to Zoom and how it has changed education. *Journal of Social Science Research, 16*(7), 33–40.

Team, G. (2021, July 7). *The distress of cumulative grief.* Georgetown Psychology. Retrieved November 15, 2023, from https://georgetownpsychology.com/2021/07/the-distress-of-cumulative-grief/

Tinder. (2021). *The future of dating is fluid.* https://www.tinderpressroom.com/futureofdating

Vasquez, A. (2021, December 11). *What's abbreviated grief? Definition + examples.* Joincake. Retrieved November 15, 2023, from https://www.joincake.com/blog/abbreviated-grief/

Williams, N. (2021). Working through COVID-19: 'Zoom' gloom and 'Zoom' fatigue. *Occupational Medicine, 71*(3), 164–164.

Wolfers, L. N., & Schneider, F. M. (2021). Using media for coping: A scoping review. *Communication Research, 48*(8), 1210–1234. https://doi.org/10.1177/0093650220939778

Wood, J. (2022). *These three charts show the global growth in online learning.* World Economic Forum. https://www.weforum.org/agenda/2022/01/online-learning-courses-reskill-skills-gap/

World Health Organization. (2021). *Fighting misinformation in the time of COVID-19, one click at a time.* https://www.who.int/news-room/feature-stories/detail/fighting-misinformation-in-the-time-of-covid-19-one-click-at-a-time

Yeung, Y. Y., & Yu, C. P. (2022). Motivating young adults to connect with nature for stress relief: A study in Taiwan during the COVID-19 pandemic. *Frontiers in Psychiatry, 13*, 922107.

Zhai, Y., & Du, X. (2020). Loss and grief amidst COVID-19: A path to adaptation and resilience. *Brain, Behavior, and Immunity, 87*, 80–81.

11 Pandemic

A Synthesised Opinion

Rakesh Verma, Sujit Verma, and Parul

The COVID-19-led pandemic not only killed millions but also shook the psychological balance of humanity from its core. The psycho-physical environment was horrifying and more than deadly. Way back in December 2019, a video clip that circulated showed health workers covered in snow-white protective gear tending to a man wearing a black suit lying prone, witnessed by passers-by. The video was reportedly from the Chinese city of Wuhan, the mother city of the virus. Some news channels dubbed Wuhan as Zombieland (McFadden, 2020). The screenshots of the spine-chilling clip are still available on the internet. Visuals of this kind were potent enough to induce fear and anxiety among the viewers. More than the virus, its fear was fatal. The lying-dead visuals provided fertile ground for the extended morbidity. Even the thought of mere infection was enough to paint the picture of impending death on the psychological retina. The fear and actual infection simultaneously ruined the body and psychological body while destabilising the mind. The shadows of death were larger than life, and fear was not an isolated emotion; instead, it was expected as a general query. It all led to a varied impact on all aspects of human beings and left thousands of questions unanswered. The source of the virus that caused the pandemic is as enigmatic as the smile of the Mona Lisa.

This synthesised chapter summarises all ten chapters at a glance, highlighting central ideas, providing thematic notes, and giving the reader an engaging experience. The chapter has been divided into ten parts, each representing a summary of each chapter.

Part 1: Psycho-social Consequences of COVID-19 across Age Groups: A Systematic Review

The psycho-social impact of COVID-19 was immense and all-pervading. Hundreds of studies were conducted to document and scientifically investigate the psycho-social effect of COVID-19. A systematic review was conducted to gather and present the findings succinctly. While keeping well with the contemporary times, the review included people of all ages, from children to veterans. After screening out irrelevant studies [in the present context], authors zeroed on 47 studies selected from a staggering 13,632 studies based on the inclusion criteria ("qualitative studies, clinical population, no consensus among reviewers, and not in the English

DOI: 10.4324/9781003454984-12

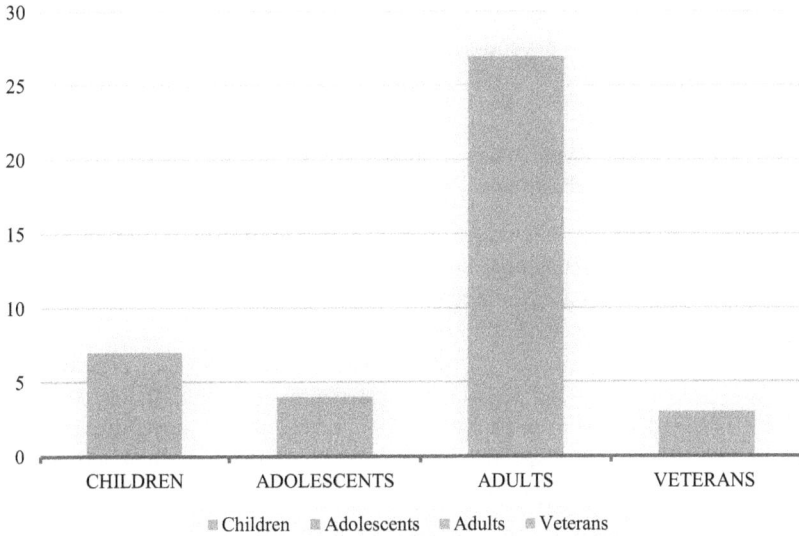

Figure 11.1 Distribution of Studies According to Age.

Data Courtesy: Respective chapter authors.

language"). The chapter rightly contains significant distribution of studies according to age (Figure 11.1).

The critical psychological issues discussed are Anxiety, Fear, Depression, Social Interaction, Irritability, OCD, Emotional and Behavioural Problems, Bedtime Resistance, Delayed Sleep Onset, Night Awakening, Parasomnia, Sleep problems, Daytime Sleep, Substance abuse, Suicide Ideation, Affect, Adjustment, Stress & Burnout, Resilience, Coping, Eating Behaviour, Job Performance, PTSD & PTS, Emotional Burden, Psychological Distress & Strain, Well-being, Occupational Stress, Physical & Mental Exhaustion, Alcohol Use, Sedentary Experience, Negative Relationship, Financial Stress, Abuse, Partner Relationship, Depersonalisation, Loneliness, Life-style, Hostility, Psycho-social Isolation, and Mental Health Expression. Additionally, factors that have psychological outcomes but not pure psychological also gained the attention of researchers, such as Meal Skipping, Quality of Life, Childcare Responsibilities, Physical Activity, Nutrition, Immuno-suppression, Religious Practices, Recreational Activities, Personal Accomplishments, Virtual Contact, Lack of Friends, Virtual Programs, and Support expression.

Out of 47 studies 15 (31.9%) examined 'Depression' as at least one of their variables, 14 (29.78%) examined 'Anxiety' as one of their variables, and 12 (25.53%) examined stress and stress-related disorders as one of their variables. The variable choices of the included studies indicate that COVID-19 is more of psychologically disorders friendly. The findings from this review suggest that to address these issues, individuals who had contracted the virus and had close encounters with the virus or those who witnessed the fury of the virus may be provided with necessary psycho-social support to erase the footprints from the cognitive beach.

Part 2: A Photovoice Exploration of Psycho-social Experiences during the COVID-19 Pandemic

The beauty of COVID-19 is that it does not discriminate. It embraces all, irrespective of age, socio-economic status, qualifications or geographical location. The second chapter focused on society's young and ambitious section, i.e., students. The researchers used a participatory research technique commonly known as Photovoice [online] for assessing and exploring the psycho-social experiences of students. Photovoice is a qualitative research technique where participants communicate their perspectives through photographs they click. "Photovoice is a process by which people can identify, and enhance their community, through a specific photographic technique" (Wang & Burris, 1997, p. 397). COVID-19 not only affected the psycho-physical profile of individuals, but it also resulted in internal mass migration, an offshoot of complete lockdown. The students who migrated (named as transition) from their institutes to their respective homes are formed samples for this study. Hostellers suddenly forced to move to their homes experienced specific changes and faced adjustment. The chapter explored the change types due to transition and subsequent adjustment issues. The selected photographs participants clicked formed the objects expressing their transitional experiences. The photographs were selected during the online live interaction sessions. In addition to the photographs, interviews, captions, photo notes, focused group discussion, and photo journals, the thematic analysis was supplemented. The chapter's 'findings and discussion' section is the most appealing section, which contains the original verbatim narrations of the participants. These narrations have emerged from the lived experiences of the participants. Some of the insights include fine-tuning with familial environs, online learning, which once seemed saviour later turned distress producer, apparel monotony, blind blanks on practical class exposure, screen phobia to screen dependence, acute deprivation of socio-academic ceremonies, ample time for self, discovering talents through hobbies, homes more than just homes, and educating parents about digital device usage. The reader gets cognitive respite from the monotony of scientific readings while sifting through this section.

Part 3: Impact and Challenges of COVID-19: A Situational Analysis

While developing the concept of 'Situational analysis' in 1957, Karl Popper might never have imagined that after more than six decades, it would be used to analyse the impact and challenges thrown up by a deadly virus (COVID-19). The ibid titled chapter has used situational analysis to pick threads of impact and challenges posed by COVID-19. The chapter had a vivid start and used an inductive writing style, encompassing academic terms, such as 'sociology of pandemic, epidemic psychology, risk society, digital risk society, unwarranted conspiracy theories, and

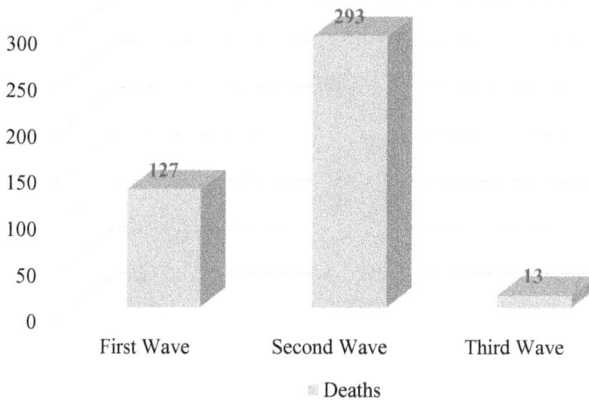

Figure 11.2 Total Reported Deaths during the Three Waves.
Data Courtesy: Respective chapter authors.

testimonial Injustice. Data from the Ballia district of Uttar Pradesh has been ana-lysed, probably due to convenience sampling. The government machinery coor-dinated and worked in tandem to tackle the pandemic by setting up testing labs and operation theatres, Paediatric Intensive Care Unit, increasing the admission facilities, sanitisation units, transportation, home delivery of medicines, and vac-cination facilities. The Integrated Covid Control and Command Centre (ICCC) was set up to monitor and coordinate among different specialised cells. Digital technology was extensively employed to aid real-time data collection, simultane-ous analysis and real-time outcomes. Both government and private health institu-tions significantly contributed to containing the spread of and treating the infection. The reported infected cases in binary numbers were indicators of the end of the respective waves. The second wave proved more deadly, where maximum casual-ties were reported (Figure 11.2).

The vaccination process was gradual and initiated on the guidelines of the state government, starting with health care workers to a vulnerable population (>60 years), 45–60 years, and then a younger lot. The two waves highlighted short-comings in public health infrastructure and essential resource allocation. For exam-ple, during the second wave, an acute shortage of oxygen was witnessed due to heavy demand. Eight oxygen generation plants were set up in Ballia to meet the surge in demand and as a preparedness measure. It was found that the mortality rate among older people (>60 years) was higher during all three waves. The male population was more affected than the female population due to several factors. The second wave affected rural areas more than the urban areas. The online data portal played a crucial role in managing the pandemic. In the concluding remarks, the authors asserted that the immunisation program helped arrest the infection and subsequent mortality trend. It was also suggested that regular updates on the por-tal were instrumental in quicker decision-making and effective implementation of public health safety measures.

Part 4: Speculated Anticipatory Anxiety of Social Interactions Post-COVID-19 Lockdown and the Reality Check

Anxiety, though a small word, has a sizeable contributory effect on psychological well-being. Anxiety is the mother of six types of psychological disorders (American Psychiatric Association, 2022). According to WHO, anxiety-based disorders are the most common psychological disorders among the world population. The leading health monitoring world agency, in its news release, claimed that the COVID-19 pandemic led (WHO, 2022). The data of the first chapter attests to these statistics, too. This chapter focused on speculated anxiety assessed through a self-designed online questionnaire containing 12 items (Equal number of positive and negative items) scored on 5-point rating scales. Again, the internet came in handy in sharing the questionnaire through social media platforms. Data collection through the internet has advantages and disadvantages; however, one of the advantages is 'wider reach'; for example, it has data from 8 Indian states. It was a live data collection type amid the pandemic, where the intensity of psychological wounds attributable to COVID-19 were fresh. An obvious advantage of this data type is the purity of its results. The findings from the survey-type study indicate that in association with mobility restrictions, self-imposed measures that grew out of self-perceived fear of infection were the top behavioural priority among the studied population. The self-perceived fear of infection stimulated anticipated anxiety and was found to be at its peak during the period of study. Additionally, the chapter highlights significant behavioural, interactional, and communication changes post-ease of mobility restrictions, which suggests the adaptive ability of humanity. Despite adjustment with changed paradigms, the chapter suggests the requirement of psychological support for those affected for general well-being.

Part 5: A Qualitative Enquiry of the Experience of Music Professionals during the COVID-19 Pandemic

SARS-Cov-2, in its world tour from late 2019 to the present day, spared no one. Music professionals were affected in several ways, too. Some gained, while some lost significantly from the gradual onslaught of COVID-19. Why is studying Indian music professionals part of this monologue? Music has been a staple for Indian cognition for 30,000 years (Vatsyayan, 1982), and music is known to improve the symptoms of mental illness (Rebecchini, 2021). The study has been designed to answer two questions, i.e., the impact of the COVID-19 pandemic on Indian music professionals and the coping mechanism employed to tide over the challenges presented by the pandemic and subsequent lockdown. The study is qualitative and based on (semi-structured) telephonic interviews of 12 music professionals who volunteered to participate during the COVID-19 onslaught. Interviews were analysed using a six-step thematic analysis method. The findings related to the first question indicate that music professionals, too, were in the grip of various psychological issues (anxiety and anger) directly impacting their mental health. They faced social issues, such as emotional intimacy [with whom they spent time during lockdown] and estrangement. The professional challenges include increased workload, financial distress, digital transformation stress, career disruption and disconnection from live audiences. The findings related to the second research question indicate that music professionals used several coping strategies to tide over the challenges imposed by COVID-19. Some coping strategies discussed include acceptance, habituation, positive life orientation, and focus on creative thinking. The study offers hope for the music industry by highlighting their plight and coping strategies. The findings can be instrumental in designing interventions for individuals associated with the music industry.

Part 6: Spiritual Dispositional Coping and Health Hardiness on Stress and Related Illnesses: Aftermath COVID-19

Spirituality is a unique human construct known only when practised. The wonder attached to the idea of spirituality is that we understand what it is but cannot define it. Nothing could define spirituality because defining it is a huge task (Ratnakar & Nair, 2012). Indians call spirituality 'addyatam' [Atam ka adhyan], i.e., study of self by knowing. Eastern practices stand tall on integrating spirituality into daily life for optimal harmonising the self. The basic tenet of spirituality is transcendence from temporal pain and sorrow. In this sense, it has taken the front seat in dealing with various psychological maladies as a potent coping mechanism.

COVID-19 has silently joined the basket of stressors already available to humankind and contributed to deteriorating mental health. Chapter 6 has addressed the role of dispositional spirituality and hardiness in coping with stress and related illnesses that have crept collectively after COVID-19. Stress-related illnesses, such as cardiovascular, respiratory, immune system dysfunction, gastrointestinal disorders, and musculoskeletal disorders are included in this study. Spiritual dispositional coping has been described in terms of attitude towards spirituality through the lenses of values and beliefs. At the same time, Kobasa's (1979) concept of health hardiness has been taken as another psychological variable. The studies done in various countries (US, Iran, Turkey, and Indonesia) in the last three decades have been cited to vindicate the role of spirituality in health hardiness. The advocacy in favour of spirituality for finding meaning and purpose in life in the event of existential crisis thrust upon humanity is well-founded and supported by appropriate literature. The spiritual practice tends to develop protective resilience against various psycho-physiological illnesses, thereby promoting total well-being. The chapter is well articulated and maintains an academic flow.

Part 7: Psychological Capital: A Determinant of the Mental Well-being of Police Personnel during COVID-19

Law enforcement agencies across the globe were among the frontline forces in the battle against the millennial fear-monger virus [COVID-19]. These agencies played roles more than they were trained for, for example, making temporary shelters for migrants (Datta et al., 2020), comforting grieving relatives, counselling the quarantines, supplying critical medicines and oxygen cylinders, supervising the cremation, creating communication channels between the infected and families. The police force was highly successful in their duty beyond the duty chart. To understand this chapter explored the role of psychological capital in maintaining mental well-being. Mitigating occupational hazards through coping and behavioural style is one of the important traits of police personnel. Kaur et al. (2013) concluded that "The personality traits and coping methods have a significant independent and interactive role in the development of high psychological stress in police persons, thus placing them at a high risk of developing psychiatric disorders". The 60 police personnel (35 males and 25 females) were examined by the Psychological Capital Questionnaire (PSQ-24) by Luthans et al. (2007), which explains Psychological Capital in four dimensions, i.e., hope, efficacy, resiliency, and optimism and Warwick Edinburgh Mental Wellbeing Scale (WEMWS-14) by Tennant et al. (2007) which consist of hedonic and eudemonic perspectives of mental health. The findings reported that police personnel were high on hope even in adverse conditions, which positively correlates with mental health. The hope factor is a significant force multiplier in dealing with stress and other related adversities posed by COVID-19-type situations. The efficacy was also higher in the participants, which, along with hope, had an additive positive effect on mental well-being. The findings of this particular study suggest that psychological capital is one of the important contributors to maintaining the mental health of police personnel in adverse situations. Indeed, it is a good read.

Part 8: Spiritual Tourism as a Panacea for COVID-19 Burnout: A Review

Spirituality is the source of comprehensive and all-pervasive comfort and the last refuse (Panacea) for individuals who perceive-cum-experience existential crisis or non-ending anxiety. Indeed, the paradigms of spirituality have provided cognitive relief to the seeker at umpteen times, which is well documented in scientific repositories. The chapter titled "Spiritual Tourism as a Panacea for COVID-19 Burnout: A Review" has attempted to review the studies that have explored the efficacy of spirituality [spiritual tourism, more specifically] in mitigating the effect of burnout that has silently slipped into the masses. Most of the studies attest to the fact that healthcare workers were the front-line victims of COVID-19-led burnout (Rossi et al., 2023), while law enforcement officers faced excessive stress during the lockdown (Khadse et al. 2020: Stogner et al., 2020). The sudden, unexpected change in lifestyle tested the coping abilities of humanity; those who were sufficiently resilient sailed through the tide of the pandemic while others faced several psychological issues, and burnout was one of them. In light of this paradigm, four research questions were framed, i.e., understanding burnout in the context of COVID-19, association of spiritual health and burnout, spiritual tourism and burnout, and spiritual tourism as an intervention technique for mitigating COVID-19-led burnout. Seven relevant articles based on arbitrarily designed inclusion criteria were included in the review. Most of the studies are on the impact of COVID-19 on the tourism industry, which specifies tourism industry was hardest hit (80% drop). The authors tried to connect the threads of findings of the identified studies. Only one of the seven studies addressed the chapter's primary variable (spiritual tourism). Spiritual tourism fostered spiritual health, which fostered resilience and strengthened the cognitive outlook. COVID-19 led to the lockdown and monotonous life by paralysing mobility, whereas spiritual tourism broke the monotony and provided the rejuvenating freshness. In the concluding remarks, the limitations of the effect of spiritual tourism have been appropriately acknowledged, and quite aptly suggested that spiritual tourism can be used as one of the alternative strategies to cope with burnout.

Part 9: Rajyoga Meditation as an Intervention Technique for Managing Negative Affect

Post-COVID-19

The coronavirus was rightly termed a dreaded avatar (Verma, 2024) that tested humanity thoroughly from all types of dimensions, such as health infrastructure, psychological resilience, law enforcement, managing fear, social paradigms, living in restricted environments, financial sector, employment issues, internal migration, meaning of life, idealness, isolation, and tourism. We were forced to explore all the possible means to counter the multifaceted effect of that dreaded avatar known as COVID-19. One of the possible ways tested by the Indian population to deal With the impact of COVID-19 was Rajyoga Meditation (RM). The RM is known to enhance positive thinking (Ramesh et al., 2013), reduce the obsession and compulsion (Mehta et al., 2020), manage physical illness (Chalageri et al., 2021), improve grey matter volume (Ramesh et al., 2021), anxiety reduction and modulation of cortisol (Kiran et al., 2017), improves essential cardiorespiratory functions (Sukhsohale & Phatak, 2012), development of emotional intelligence competencies (Singh, 2021) and improvement in physiological and psychological general well-being (Sukhsohale et al., 2012). The scientific literature has sufficient evidence to vindicate the efficacy of RM in managing the overall well-being of human beings. Against this backdrop, to attest to the efficacy of RM, 87 (12 male) participants from Vipul World Society Gurugram, Haryana (India) were administered RM for eight weeks. In this quasi-experimental pre-post research design, the sample was assessed for the impact of RM on negative affect using 88-state questionnaires. The results showed a significant decrease in the negative affect mean score of the participant post-RM intervention. In the concluding statement, the authors suggested that RM can be an effective intervention strategy to manage psychological well-being if practised regularly under expert supervision.

Part 10: A Critical Study: The Transactional Concept of Coping through Electronic Media during the COVID-19 Pandemic

Social media, a highly influential offshoot of electronic media (EM), has seemed to erase the term and its core idea commonly known as the 'generation gap' introduced by John Poppy in 1967. Though media has played one of the most critical roles of opinion managers since its inception, in current affairs, EM has donned roles beyond its expected scope. EM was the most common source of information during the pandemic, helping mitigate psychological concerns (Bilal et al., 2020) and break misconceptions and myths (Srivastava et al., 2018). Media has an essential role in coping with psychological disorders symptoms (Naslund et al., 2020) and treatment of mental disorders (Haidt & Allen, 2020), and on the other EM is leading to specialised stress (Huff, 2022). With its tremendous growth, EM has extended the basic definition of the transactional concept, where one individual transacts with several people simultaneously and communicates accordingly. EM was the only option available during the COVID-19 for communication beyond the four walls of houses. EM, especially social media, acted as a vent for expression and interpersonal interaction, a kind of digital catharsis, one of its kind of coping. One example that vindicates the role of EM during the pandemic is that of Tinder dating application. The application recorded around 3 billion swipes in a single day in March 2020 (Molla, 2021). Similar trends were observed on online platforms, such as counselling, academics, music, learning, video, blogging, and news. Such a vast population shift towards the virtual world is a testament to the use of EM for beating the isolation blues.

In conclusion, the EM connected grieving families, comforted and connected friends, provided psychological interventions, offered choices of entertainment, familiarised students and teachers with virtual teaching-learning systems, webinars replaced seminar norms, revolutionised the banking and payment systems (Unified Payment Interface) and provided an alternate source of earnings. Despite pandemic-led hardship, the EM was the only hope where humanity could find comfort in its lap.

Acknowledgement

We would like to acknowledge all the authors for their high-quality content, which was the basis for this piece. It would be wrong if we did not express our deepest gratitude to Dr Rajesh Verma for motivating us to summarise the book and for providing regular feedback and insight while preparing this manuscript.

References

American Psychiatric Association. (2022). *Anxiety disorders. Diagnostic and statistical manual of mental disorders. Text revision* (5th ed., pp. 215–231). Author.
Bilal, L. F., Bashir, M. F., Komal, B., & Tan, D. (2020). Role of electronic media in mitigating the psychological impacts of novel coronavirus (COVID-19). *Psychiatry Research, 289*, 113041. https://doi.org/10.1016/j.psychres.2020.113041
Chalageri, E., Vishwakarma, G., Ranjan, R. L., Govindaraj, R., & Chhabra, H. S. (2021). Effect of Rāja Yoga meditation on psychological and functional outcomes in spinal cord injury patients. *International Journal of Yoga, 14*(1), 36–42. https://doi.org/10.4103/ijoy.IJOY_68_20
Datta, T., Ray, S., & Dawa, M. (2020, May). Re-imagining the role of the police in COVID-19 times. *UNICEF.* https://www.unicef.org/india/stories/re-imagining-role-police-covid-19-times

Haidt, J., & Allen, N. (2020). Scrutinising the effects of digital technology on mental health. *Nature, 578*(7794), 226–227. https://doi.org/10.1038/d41586-020-00296-x

Huff, C. (2022). Media overload is hurting our mental health. Here are ways to manage headline stress. *Monitor on Psychology, 53*(8). https://www.apa.org/monitor/2022/11/strain-media-overload

Kaur, R., Chodagiri, V. K., & Reddi, N. K. (2013). A psychological study of stress, personality and coping in police personnel. *Indian Journal of Psychological Medicine, 35*(2), 141–147. https://doi.org/10.4103/0253-7176.116240

Khadse, P. A., Gowda, G. S., Ganjekar, S., Desai, G., & Murthy, P. (2020). Mental health impact of COVID-19 on police personnel in India. *Indian Journal of Psychological Medicine, 42*(6), 580–582. https://doi.org/10.1177/0253717620963345

Kiran, U., Ladha, S., Makhija, N., Kapoor, P. M., Choudhury, M., Das, S., Gharde, P., Malik, V., & Airan, B. (2017). The role of Rajyoga meditation for modulation of anxiety and serum cortisol in patients undergoing coronary artery bypass surgery: A prospective randomised control study. *Annals of Cardiac Anaesthesia, 20*(2), 158–162. https://doi.org/10.4103/aca.ACA_32_17

Kobasa, S. C. (1979). Stressful life events, personality, and health – Inquiry into hardiness. *Journal of Personality and Social Psychology, 37*(1), 1–11. https://doi.org/10.1037/0022-3514.37.1

Luthans, F., Avolio, B. J., & Avey, J. B. (2007). *Psychological capital questionnaire*. New York: Mind Garden Inc.

McFadden, B (2020, January 24). Coronavirus: Infected people seen 'dead in streets' in Chinese city dubbed 'Zombieland'. *Mirror*. https://www.mirror.co.uk/news/world-news/infected-people-seen-dead-streets-21347952

Mehta, K., Mehta, S., Chalana, H., Singh, H., & Thaman, R. G. (2020). Effectiveness of Rajyoga Meditation as an adjunct to first-line treatment in patients with obsessive-compulsive disorder. *Indian Journal of Psychiatry, 62*(6), 684–689. https://doi.org/10.4103/psychiatry.IndianJPsychiatry_401_19

Molla, R. (2021, March 25). Tinder data shows how pandemic dating was even weirder than regular dating. *Technology*. https://www.vox.com/recode/22348298/tinder-data-video-online-dating-pandemic

Naslund, J. A., Bondre, A., Torous, J., & Aschbrenner, K. A. (2020). Social media and mental health: Benefits, risks, and opportunities for research and practice. *Journal of Technology in Behavioral Science, 5*(3), 245–257. https://doi.org/10.1007/s41347-020-00134-x

Ramesh, B. M. G., Kadavigere, R., Koteshwara, P., Sathian, B., & Rai, K. S. (2021). Rajyoga meditation experience induces enhanced positive thoughts and alters grey matter volume of brain regions: A Cross-sectional Study. *Mindfulness, 12*, 1659–1671. https://doi.org/10.1007/s12671-021-01630-8

Ramesh, M. G., Sathian, B., Sinu, E., & Kiranmai, S. R. (2013). Efficacy of Rajayoga meditation on positive thinking: An index for self-satisfaction and happiness in life. *Journal of Clinical and Diagnostic Research: JCDR, 7*(10), 2265–2267. https://doi.org/10.7860/JCDR/2013/5889.3488

Ratnakar, R., & Nair, S. (2012). A review of scientific research on spirituality. *Business Perspectives and Research, 1*, 1–12. https://www 10.1177/2278533720120101

Rebecchini, L. (2021). Music, mental health, and immunity. *Brain, Behavior, & Immunity – Health, 18*, 100374. https://doi.org/10.1016/j.bbih.2021.100374

Rossi, M. F., Gualano, M. R., Magnavita, N., Moscato, U., Santoro, P. E., & Borrelli, I. (2023). Coping with burnout and the impact of the COVID-19 pandemic on workers' mental health: A systematic review. *Frontiers in Psychiatry, 14,* 1139260. https://doi.org/10.3389/fpsyt.2023.1139260

Singh, P. (2021). Emotional intelligence competencies developed through raja yoga meditation: A study of women in the national capital region of India. *The Journal of Contemporary Issues in Business and Government, 27,* 791–804.

Srivastava, K., Chaudhury, S., Bhat, P. S., & Mujawar, S. (2018). Media and mental health. *Industrial Psychiatry Journal, 27*(1), 1–5. https://doi.org/10.4103/ipj.ipj_73_18

Stogner, J., Miller, B. L., & McLean, K. (2020). Police stress, mental health, and resiliency during the COVID-19 pandemic. *American Journal of Criminal Justice, 45*(4), 718–730. https://doi.org/10.1007/s12103-020-09548-y

Sukhsohale, N. D., & Phatak, M. S. (2012). Effect of short-term and long-term Brahmakumaris Rajayoga meditation on physiological variables. *Indian Journal of Physiological Pharmacology, 56*(4), 388–392. PMID: 23781660.

Sukhsohale, N. D., Phatak, M. S., Sukhsohale, S. D., & Agrawal, S. B. (2012). Does Raja Yoga meditation brings out physiological and psychological general well-being among practitioners of it. *International Journal of Collaborative Research on Internal Medicine and Public Health, 4*(12).

Tennant, R., Hiller, L., Fishwick, R., Platt, S., Joseph, S., Weich, S., & Stewart-Brown, S. (2007). The Warwick-Edinburgh mental well-being scale (WEMWBS): Development and UK Validation. *Health and Quality of Life Outcomes, 5*(1), 1–13.

Verma, R. (2024). Coronavirus: The dreaded avatar that surprised humanity. In R. Verma, U. Uzaina, S. Manickam, T. Singh, & G. Tiwari (Eds.), *Exploring the psycho-social impact of COVID-19: Global perspectives on behaviour, interventions and future directions* (pp. 1–18). New York: Routledge. https://www.routledge.com/Exploring-the-Psycho-Social-Impact-of-COVID-19-Global-Perspectives-on-Behaviour/Verma-Uzaina-Manickam-Singh-Tiwari/p/book/9781003357209

Vatsyayan, K. (1982). *Dance in Indian painting.* India: Abhinav Publications.World Health Organisation. (2022, March 02). Wake-up call to all countries to step up mental health services and support. COVID-19 pandemic triggers 25% increase in prevalence of anxiety and depression worldwide (who.int).

Wang, C., & Burris, M. A. (1997). Photovoice: Concept, methodology, and use for participatory needs assessment. *Health Education & Behavior, 24*(3), 369–387. https://doi.org/10.1177/109019819702400309

Index

For Product Safety Concerns and Information please contact our EU
representative GPSR@taylorandfrancis.com
Taylor & Francis Verlag GmbH, Kaufingerstraße 24, 80331 München, Germany

www.ingramcontent.com/pod-product-compliance
Lightning Source LLC
Chambersburg PA
CBHW060258220326
41598CB00027B/4158